CHINA'S
LAST NOMADS

Studies on Modern China

Studies on Modern China

CHINA'S
LAST NOMADS
The History and Culture of China's Kazaks

LINDA BENSON AND INGVAR SVANBERG

An East Gate Book

M.E. Sharpe
Armonk, New York
London, England

An East Gate Book

Copyright © 1998 by M. E. Sharpe, Inc.

Photo section starts after page 170. Photos on the first four pages are taken from
Xinjiang Sangu Geming (Xinjiang's Three District Revolution).
Urumqi: Xinjiang Meishu Sheying Chubanshe, 1994.

Library of Congress Cataloging-in-Publication Data

Benson, Linda.
China's last Nomads : the history and culture of China's
Kazaks / Linda Benson and Ingvar Svanberg.
p.   cm.—(Studies on modern China)
Includes bibliographical references.
ISBN 1-56324-781-X (cloth : alk. paper).—
ISBN 1-56324-782-8 (pbk. : alk. paper)
1. Kazakhs—China—History—20th century.   2. Sinkiang Uighur
Autonomous Region (China)—Ethnic relations.
I. Svanberg, Ingvar, 1953–   . II. Series.
DS731.K38B46   1997
952′.00494345—dc21   97-45582
CIP
Printed in the United States of America

Contents

Preface

When we first began our research on China's Kazak population, well over a decade ago, little had been written on specific minority populations in China—with the notable exception of the Tibetans and Mongols, each of which has been the subject of considerable scholarly work. Our first effort consisted of an edited collection of essays on the Kazaks, published in Sweden in 1988. It was based both on fieldwork undertaken in 1986 and on extensive archival research in such disparate places as England, the former West Germany, the United States, Taiwan, Hong Kong, and Sweden. Ten years later, two developments have made a new study both feasible and necessary. First, the 1991 collapse of the Soviet Union led to the emergence of a new political order in Central Asia. While the effects of the dissolution of the USSR are still unfolding, for the first time in modern history, Central Eurasian peoples like the Kazaks have their own independent states, allowing them to begin a reexamination of their history and culture. The extent of the impact of this extraordinary event on China's Kazaks, most of whom live in districts that share a border with the newly independent state of Kazakstan, is assessed in the final chapter of this book.

A second factor in our decision to revisit the history and culture of China's Kazaks was the People's Republic of China's (PRC) decision to allow better access to the national archives, making new sources of information available and allowing a more extensive examination of the historic development of the Kazaks as a national minority. Both the new political reality of Kazakstan's presence on the Chinese border and new archival sources inform this study of the Kazak experience inside China's borders.

Just as we were completing our manuscript, in February 1997, the most serious ethnic disturbance in Xinjiang since 1949 occurred in Yining, the prefectural capital of the largest Kazak area in China.

Although the complete story of what happened there may not be known for some time, this event dramatically emphasizes the heightened sense of nationalism in China's far northwest.

The authors owe much to many, not all of whom can be acknowledged here. Certainly, without the friendship, hospitality, and inspiration of many Kazaks, this book would not have been written, and we are grateful to Kazaks in China as well as among the Kazak diaspora in Turkey and Europe for their assistance and inspiration. Mr. Arslan Tosun (Germany), Mr. Halife Altay (Turkey), and Mr. Cengizhan Aksakal (Sweden) provided guidance and insight, as did American scholars such as Professor Frank Bessac and Professor A. Doak Barnett, both of whom met with the Kazaks during the tumultuous years of the 1940s.

Financial support for Ingvar Svanberg came from the Swedish Council for Social Research (94–0162) and from the Swedish Council for Research in the Humanities and Social Sciences (F 147/94). In addition, the collegial atmosphere of the Department of East European Studies and the Department of the History of Religions at Uppsala University provided him with much appreciated support as he completed work on parts of the manuscript. The isolated Faroe Islands and friends there offered a convivial setting conducive to writing and research. To all of these institutions and individuals, Ingvar Svanberg extends his thanks and appreciation.

Linda Benson received financial support from Oakland University's research committee, which provided a faculty fellowship, making possible her return to Xinjiang in 1996. A sabbatical leave provided her the time to write and travel. For both forms of assistance, she extends her thanks. Appreciation is also due to the hardworking and efficient staff of the Second Historical Archives in Nanjing, where some materials pertaining to the Guomindang's policy in Xinjiang were made available. A special word of gratitude is due Mr. Garvin Davenport, currently a doctoral student at the University of Illinois, whose help and good company in Nanjing were much appreciated. The Shanghai Public Library proved a useful repository, and the staff were quite efficient and helpful. Although it is not appropriate to name them here, colleagues in Hong Kong, Taiwan, Australia, Nanjing, Shanghai, Beijing, and Xinjiang were generous with their knowledge and their time. As is always the case, however, the conclusions presented in this book are solely the responsibility of the authors, not of these individuals. Linda Benson also acknowledges with love and gratitude the ongoing support and encouragement of her extended family—the Benson, Maines, Wu, and Moran, clans of the United States and Taiwan. Above all, she extends her thanks to her husband, David Maines, who, on his first visit to China, gamely agreed to journey across the Gobi Desert to northwestern China, providing good company and wise counsel while crammed into the back of crowded buses, taxis, and planes and enduring what must have seemed interminable visits to bookstores and libraries. Given the circumstances, thanks alone are inadequate; but he, hopefully, understands how much his support was and is appreciated.

In the United States and Sweden, colleagues who have contributed in various ways to the authors' ongoing study of Xinjiang include Dorothy Borei, Garvin Davenport, Dru Gladney, Gunnar Jarring, Dolkun Kamberi, Jonathan Lipman, Justin Rudelson, and Stanley Toops, geographer par excellence of the Xinjiang region. Our publisher, Douglas Merwin, editor, Mai Cota, copyeditor Will Moore, and project editor Angela Piliouras, were patient as we made final revisions, and we are grateful for their support. To all these individuals and to the departments and institutions mentioned above, we both extend our thanks.

A Note on Romanization

We have used the *Hanyu pinyin* system of romanization for most Chinese names and words. Choosing a system for place-names and individuals in Xinjiang is more problematic, as there is no agreement on the most appropriate form for romanized Kazak or Uyghur. Therefore, we have opted for those forms that we believe are most accessible to an English language–reading audience. In general, place-names that have an accepted English rendering are spelled in that form—for example, Kashgar and Khotan (instead of the Chinese forms, *Kashi* and *Hetian*). Less familiar places in Xinjiang that have a Chinese name appear in the *pinyin* system, but are followed by the locally used Turkic form in parentheses—for example, Yining [Gulja] and Hami [Komul]. Personal names of Turkic people are rendered in modified modern Turkish, without diacritical marks, thus avoiding clumsy "sinified" forms, such as the nearly indecipherable Halibaike for Ali Beg Hakim. Kazak terms are spelled according to a modified form of the system in Menges, *Philologiae Turicicae Fundamenta* (1959), without diacritical marks. Russian words are transliterated according to the system in Comrie, *The World's Major Languages* (1987).

Abbreviations and Measurements

List of Abbreviations

CCP   Chinese Communist Party
CPPCC   Chinese People's Political Consultative Conference
GMD   Guomindang (Kuomintang or Nationalist Party)
NCNA   New China News Agency (Xinhua)
OSS   Office of Strategic Services
PCC   Production and Construction Corp
PLA   People's Liberation Army
PRC   People's Republic of China

List of Abbreviations in Sources

CB   Current Background
FBIS   Foreign Broadcast Information Service
FBIS-CHI   Foreign Broadcast Information Service-China
SCMM   Survey of China Mainland Magazines
SCMP   Survey of China Mainland Press
JPRS   Joint Publications Research Service
JPRS-CAR   Joint Publications Research Service-Central Asian Review
JMJP   People's Daily [originally Jen Min Jih Pao]
SWB/FE   Summary of World Broadcasts/Far East

Measurements

1 mu = .0667 hectares or, 1/6 of an acre
1 catty = 0.604 kilograms or, 1.33 lb.
1 jin = 0.5 kilograms or, 1.1 lb.

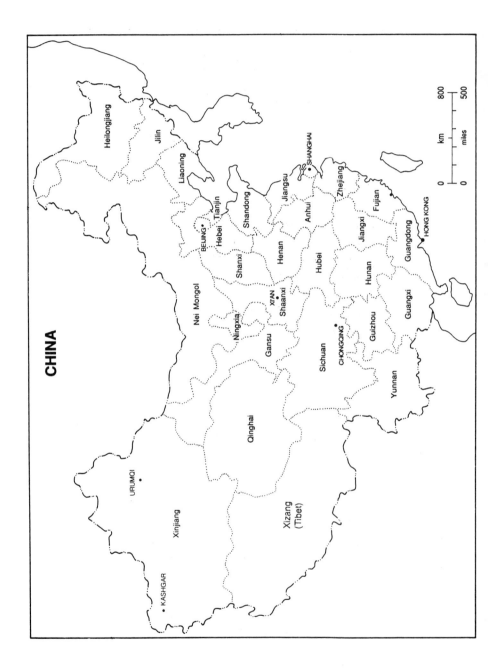

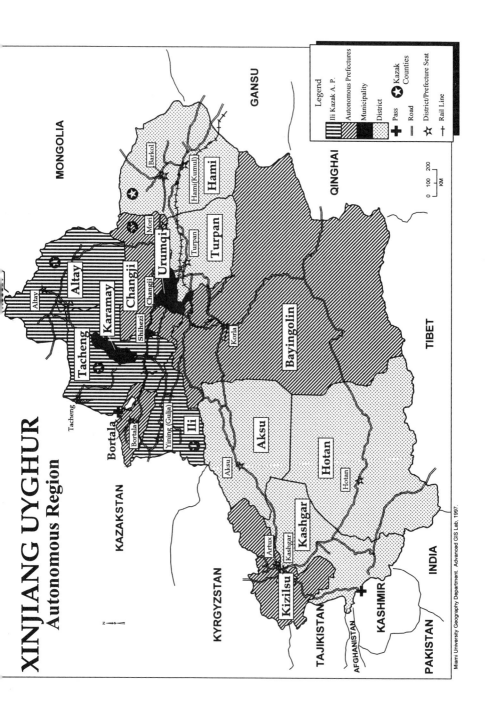

XINJIANG UYGHUR
Autonomous Region

MONGOLIA

GANSU

QINGHAI

TIBET

KAZAKSTAN

KYRGYZSTAN

TAJIKISTAN

AFGHANISTAN

KASHMIR

INDIA

PAKISTAN

Barkol

Hami(Kumul)

Hami

Mori

Turpan

Turpan

Urumqi

Changji

Changji

Altay

Altay

Karamay

Shihezi

Tacheng

Tacheng

Korla

Bayingolin

Bortala

Bortala

Yining (Gulja)

Ili

Aksu

Aksu

Hotan

Hotan

Kashgar

Kashgar

Artux

Kizilsu

Legend

Ili Kazak A. P.

Autonomous Prefectures

Municipality

District

Kazak Counties

Pass

Road

District/Prefecture Seat

Rail Line

0   100   200

KM

Miami University Geography Department. Advanced GIS Lab, 1997.

CHINA'S
LAST NOMADS

Introduction

For 150 years, Central Asian peoples like the Kazaks were the reluctant subjects of powerful neighboring empires, their lands being added to the expanding territories of Russia and China through a series of conquests in the nineteenth century. From the west, czarist armies swept eastwards across the Urals, conquering Central Asian khanates and acquiring vast stretches of the Kazak steppe. From the east, the Manchu rulers of China asserted their authority over the grasslands of today's Xinjiang-Uyghur Autonomous Region—the easternmost geographical extension of the Central Eurasian steppes. China's military conquest led to the formal incorporation of an area once known as Eastern Turkestan into the Qing dynasty's empire in 1884, making it a province for the first time in China's history. In the twentieth century, the revolutionary successor states of both empires maintained their claims over Central Eurasia, dividing people like the Kazaks with new international borders, separating not only clans but also individual families on either side of the Sino-Soviet frontier.

The imposition of communist rule over traditionally nomadic peoples like the Kazaks was accomplished despite their resistance to such revolutionary change. Thereafter, both the Soviet and Chinese governments carefully controlled access to Kazak lands, with the result that scholars interested in Kazak history and culture have had to glean what they could from government-generated statistics or from scholarly accounts heavily dominated by Marxist rhetoric. Although isolation and government controls did not totally suppress research, political circumstances nonetheless meant that the study of this region was greatly restricted.

In 1991, the Central Eurasian regions of the USSR abruptly became independent; for the first time in this century, Muslim peoples like the Kazaks, Uzbeks, and Kirghiz governed their own states—a dramatic change that immediately raised concerns for Russia, the former Soviet republics, and the government of the neighboring People's Republic of

China and that subsequently has demanded different approaches to regional and international relations. The reconfiguration of power in Central Eurasia has also brought into focus the past circumstances and present fate of the ethnic minority populations of both former empires, increasing international awareness of minorities whose history and culture have remained relatively unknown in the West. As is the case in many troubled nation-states today, minorities in China and Russia have been viewed as troublesome, even rebellious citizens, whose insistence on following traditional religious and cultural practices and whose rejection of the state's national agendas has resulted in government suppression and repression. Clearly, neither the former nor present communist systems ruling in Central Eurasia have discovered workable solutions to the problematic existence of minority populations within their borders.

This book examines the experience of Kazaks as a minority population in China, focusing on the twentieth century and examining the Kazak experience in the multiethnic region of Xinjiang. It is not intended to be predictive, for that would be a precarious business given the dramatic and rapid changes occurring in East and Central Asia. Nor is it meant to be exhaustive on all aspects of Kazak life. Instead, this work is intended to provide an account of the history and circumstances of the Kazaks in China in the twentieth century, a period that saw them separated from Kazaks in the USSR, introduced to communism, and, most recently, allowed to return to the family-owned flocks and herds that constituted the local Kazak economy prior to 1949. As demonstrated in the chapters that follow, the days in which Kazaks of the northwest pursued the independent lifestyle of their ancestors are gone. Their future will be shaped by increasing interaction with the growing number of Han Chinese residents of China's great northwest, and by Chinese policies that determine patterns of land and water use as well as market exchange. Understanding past Kazak experience in China documents what is being lost and suggests a range of possibilities for this ethnic minority in the twenty-first century.

Sources

In writing this book, we are drawing on years of interest in and travel to the Xinjiang region, where the majority of China's Kazaks have lived for over 200 years. Between us we have examined Russian and

Chinese sources as well as the small amount of literature available to us in Turkish and Kazak. Those secondary sources in English and other European languages used in the preparation of our book are listed in the bibliography. While this body of work is considerable, it is important to note that the sources for research on Kazak history—both printed and oral—continue to present problems to the researcher. The reader must bear in mind that this region was among the last areas of China to open to the outside world and that Chinese sensitivity over minority affairs continues to limit access to Chinese archival sources and to impose restrictions on fieldwork. Many of the available sources reflect these political limitations. In the circumstances, all materials have been used with caution. We hope that we have managed to avoid being drawn into an overreliance on government-generated documents, while not discounting some of the excellent work by both Soviet-Russian and Chinese scholars concerned with the history and culture of the Kazak people. We have also used, as extensively as restrictions have allowed, interviews with Kazaks and other Muslim peoples from the area, both current residents and émigrés who are now part of a world-wide Kazak diaspora. In recent years, Chinese publications on language, culture, and history have provided interesting new materials that, despite being colored by the official Communist Party line, nonetheless contribute to the current scholarship on China's Kazaks. If the current policy of "opening up to the outside world" is allowed to continue in Xinjiang, it is to be hoped that future studies will be able to investigate more thoroughly some of the many issues raised in the present volume.

This study joins a body of work on the Kazaks that began nearly two centuries ago. Much of this scholarship concerns Kazaks of the Russian sphere. Among the pioneers researching Kazak history were the nineteenth-century scholars Aleksis Levshin and Vilhelm Radlov, whose works, published in French and German, referred primarily to the Kazaks of the Russian empire. During the same period, the Kazak scholar Chokan Chingisovich Valikhanov compiled invaluable information on Kazak cultural history and ethnography. Although he was Russian-educated and served as an officer in the czarist military, his insight into Kazak traditions was unequaled by his contemporaries. Still valuable, early twentieth-century accounts of Kazak life were written by the German ethnographer Richard Karutz and the French ethnographer Joseph Castagné.

After the October Revolution of 1917, the access of European or American scholars to Soviet Central Asia was severely restricted. However, in 1936, American anthropologist Alfred E. Hudson had the opportunity to conduct fieldwork on the social organization of the Kazaks in the USSR. His work, *Kazak Social Structure* (1938), is still regarded as a minor classic. Subsequently, several American and European scholars compiled works on Kazak ethnography and social organization with the assistance of earlier written sources and Soviet scholarly research. Examples of this type of work can be seen in the writings of George P. Murdock and C. Daryll Forde. In the 1960s, the work of Russian scholar Valentin Riasanovsky (1965) added to the literature on Kazaks in the USSR, as did the important books and articles of Lawrence Krader (1955, 1962, 1963) and Elizabeth Bacon (1958, 1966). In Europe, Viktor Dingelstedt published his study on Kazak social organization at around the same time. Martha Brill Olcott published a 1987 political history of the Kazaks in the USSR, followed in recent years by studies of the newly independent states of the Commonwealth of Independent States (CIS). All of these works focus on the Kazaks of the USSR, and few mention the Kazak groups in China.

Soviet literature on Kazak history and culture is very extensive. A general indication of the quantity of such work can be gleaned from the bibliographies of the various works by Krader and Bacon. Russian-language items written prior to the 1991 dissolution of the USSR remain among the most valuable sources on a wide range of topics related to Kazak language, cultural practices, and social organization. Since 1991, interest in Central Eurasia and in the Kazaks of the former Soviet Union has grown worldwide. Though relatively few new works dealing with the specific histories of Central Eurasia have emerged thus far, this lack will no doubt be remedied in the near future as opportunities expand for research and travel into these once-closed regions.

In contrast, writing on minorities in China has remained a neglected enterprise. While scattered works in English and Chinese surveyed China's northwestern region prior to 1949, most focused on the area's political situation, rather than on its specific minority populations. Among the few scholars to publish articles in the 1960s on the Kazaks of Xinjiang are Toru Saguchi and Frank Bessac, the latter basing his articles on personal experiences among the Kazaks during the winter of 1949–50. After Bessac's historic visit, American and European access ended, so that only a handful of studies on the isolated Kazaks have since appeared in Western languages.

Although the past decade has seen the publication of a few studies breaking new ground on issues of ethnicity, nationalism, and identity in China, histories of the various "national minorities"—as they are called in the PRC—have yet to be written. Recent American works by Stevan Harrell (1995), William Jankowiak, Jonathan Lipman, Dru Gladney, Charles McKhann, and Justin Rudelson provide anthropological studies that examine the status and circumstances of minority groups such as the Yi, the Mongols (of Inner Mongolia), the Hui, the Naxi, and the Uyghur. With the exception of Gladney's study of the Hui (1990), however, this work has been in the form of book chapters rather than book-length studies. In China, works by Kazak scholar Niqmet Manjani (1987) and Han Chinese author Su Beihai (1989) as well as government-sponsored histories of the Kazaks and other northwestern Muslim peoples augment a growing field of research inside and beyond China's borders on individual minority groups—but much exciting work remains ahead.

The present book on Kazak history and culture thus joins a small but growing literature on minorities in China. Building on the authors' previous research and their repeated visits to the Xinjiang region over the past fifteen years, it also draws on those archival resources currently available in China and Taiwan. It seeks to provide an account of Kazak history in China, giving particular emphasis to those aspects that have shaped this group's identity in ways that differ from the majority of the Kazak population just across the border. The Kazak response to China's efforts at modifying and controlling Kazak cultural expression is an important facet of their new identity as a minority nationality in a powerful, modernizing Han Chinese state.

Contemporary Distribution of the Kazak People

As late as the early twentieth century, the Kazaks were still referred to by a variety of names spelled in a variety of ways: the Kirghiz, Kirghiz-Kazaks, Kirghiz Kaissaks, or Kazak-Kirghiz. One of the functions of these names was to differentiate them from the Cossacks, who were a military unit under the Russian czar and not a Central Asian people at all. The people we today call the Kirghiz (now romanized as "Kyrgyz" in the new republic of Kyrgyzstan) were called the Kara-

Table I.1

Kazak Populations, 1990

Country	Population
Kazakstan	6,534,616
China	1,111,718
Uzbekistan	808,227
Russia	784,000
Karakalpakstan	319,000
Mongolia	137,000
Turkmenistan	87,802
Kyrgyzstan	37,318
Tajikistan	11,376
Turkey	5,000
Western Europe	2,000
Total	9,831,057

Kirghiz [Black Kirghiz] or the "mountain" Kirghiz in earlier literature. In 1926, the Soviet Union officially introduced the ethnonym "КАЗАХ" [Kazakh] in keeping with the Soviet policy of officially recognizing names used by the ethnic groups themselves. As a result, the name "Kazakh" gained international recognition as the correct term for identifying this Turkic Muslim nomadic people. Here, we follow Kazakstan's practice, using the spelling "Kazak," rather than the Russian-language-based form, "Kazakh."

The world's total Kazak population is approximately 10 million, with the largest numbers concentrated in Kazakstan, China, Uzbekistan, and Russia, summarized in Table I.1. By far the largest concentration of Kazaks is in the Republic of Kazakstan, which became independent of Soviet control in December 1991. The last Soviet census (in 1989) placed the Kazak population in the USSR at 8,135,818, with 6.1 million living in the Kazak Soviet republic; a sizable number also lived in Russia, especially in and near the cities of Astrakhan, Saratov, Orenburg, and Omsk, with another concentration in the Russian Altay region. Over the past twenty-five years, there has been a steady migration of Kazaks from other areas of the USSR into Kazakstan. Since 1991, the numbers of new immigrants jumped as Kazaks from Mongolia, China, Iran, and former Soviet republics were welcomed by the new government. Returning Kazaks, plus a high

Kazak birthrate, has meant that an increasing percentage of Kazakstan's population is ethnic Kazak: In 1993 they constituted 43.2 percent of the population, while the percentage of Russians decreased to 36.4 percent.[1]

Outside of the former USSR, there is a relatively long-established Kazak community in Mongolia. According to the 1989 Mongolian census, 137,000 Kazaks lived there, many with relatives across the border in China. They were concentrated in the Bayan-Ölgii district (83,000) and the Kentei and Dornod districts (4,300). Urban Kazaks live in the far-western district of Hovd (12,000) and in Selenge and Ulan Bator (9,100). Many Kazaks in Mongolia still make their living from animal husbandry, while some have chosen to work in Mongolia's mining industry. As a result of the changes and economic disruptions in Mongolia after 1990, an estimated 5,000 Kazak families left for Kazakstan where they were granted land and other assistance to help them settle. By the mid-1990s, however, such migrations appeared to have halted, as expectations of a new life in Kazakstan were not met (for further discussion of Kazakstan, see chapter 7).[2]

Small Kazak populations have also lived in Afghanistan and Iran. Particularly in the late 1920s, thousands of Kazaks fled into northern Afghanistan, where they settled mainly in towns, living among the poorest strata of society. Estimates of their numbers have varied: Soviet figures in 1962 reported some 3,000 Kazaks in Afghanistan, while an American estimate in 1978 put this population at 20,000. After Soviet troops entered the region in 1978, Kazaks were among the many refugees fleeing the country, facing uncertain futures in Turkey and western Europe. Some Kazaks reportedly remained and still live in the region of Khanabad, with smaller numbers in Andkhui and around Herat.[3] Iran's Kazak population also dates mainly from the early part of the twentieth century, when refugees from Kazakstan settled in the area of Behshahr and Gorgan, along the Caspian Sea. In 1968, their population was estimated at 400 families.[4] Official contacts between these foreign Kazak communities and Kazakstani authorities have been established, and the Kazakstani government is permitting their repatriation.[5]

Kazak populations outside the former USSR, such as those mentioned above, have been little studied. An exception is the Kazaks of Turkey, whose lives are documented in a 1989 monograph by Ingvar Svanberg. These are primarily descendants of Kazaks from China, given refuge by the Turkish government in the late 1940s and early 1950s. Originally settled in rural areas, many moved to urban environs in the 1960s and 1970s. Today, they live in segregated settlements in Istanbul, Ankara, Izmir, and Adana. Most are employed in the manufacture of leather goods, but some have shifted to work in plastics factories. Some remain in the original Kazak settlements in Salihli, Konya, Nigde, and Sultanhani.[6]

Beginning in the 1960s, Kazaks have also migrated in small numbers to industrialized countries of the West. Many arrived to work as laborers in European cities. By the 1990s, small Kazak enclaves had been established in Germany, France, and Sweden, with smaller numbers in Austria, the Netherlands, Belgium, and Norway. Small numbers of Kazaks are also scattered elsewhere around the world. Since the 1970s, Kazak groups have established themselves in the Middle East and now live in the various countries of the Arabian Peninsula. A much smaller number has arrived in the United States, primarily from among the Kazaks of Turkey. Others live in Pakistan and Taiwan.[7] In the mid-1990s, many members of the Kazak diaspora have sought contact with Kazakstan, and those who enjoy prosperity in their adoptive states have begun to invest in a small way in Kazakstan's still-troubled economy.

China's population of an estimated 1.2 million Kazaks is the largest outside of the Republic of Kazakstan. Concentrated in the Xinjiang-Uyghur Autonomous Region, the majority of Kazaks live in areas contiguous with the Kazakstani border, which separates not only clans but individual families. Other Kazaks in China live in the provinces of Gansu and Qinghai, where autonomous local-level governments have been established for them, in keeping with the People's Republic of China's laws on autonomy for minority nationalities. In examining the history and culture of the Kazaks, we begin with a discussion of the geographic and cultural setting in which China's Kazak minority has lived for several centuries and then turn in successive chapters to their history and present status as one of China's national minorities.

— 1 —

The Kazaks of Northwestern China: The Physical and Cultural Setting

The vast majority of China's Kazaks live in Xinjiang, the single largest administrative unit in the People's Republic of China (PRC). Covering a sixth of China, this geographically diverse territory was officially renamed the Xinjiang-Uyghur Autonomous Region in 1955 in recognition of its single most populous group, the Uyghurs. Second in terms of population are the Kazaks, who began moving into Xinjiang in the eighteenth century, establishing themselves on pastures in the central and northern mountain ranges of the territory. The sedentary Uyghurs traditionally populated the oasis cities, which once served the Silk Road, a trade artery that linked China to the Middle East and Europe for some two thousand years. The differing requirements of the Kazak and Uyghur livelihoods, combined with the varied topography of the Xinjiang region and a relatively sparse population, allowed both nomadic and sedentary peoples to live side by side in relative harmony. Periodically, their shared religious beliefs as well as a shared Turkic heritage drew them together in popularly supported movements against local Chinese administrations. Thus, a key to understanding the history of northwestern China and its Kazak people is Xinjiang's physical and human geography—the study of which sets the stage for an examination of the Kazaks today and their current relations with the other inhabitants of the vast Xinjiang region.

Xinjiang's Geography

As China's single largest administrative region, Xinjiang covers 1,646,000 square kilometers, which is approximately one-sixth of Chinese territory. The regional capital of Urumqi is nearly 3,000 kilometers from the national capital at Beijing; even the nearest provincial capital, Xining in the neighboring province of Qinghai, is a considerable distance away at 1,590 kilometers. The region's distance from what is sometimes referred to as China proper has been one barrier to its integration with the Chinese state, but natural barriers have been equally effective in separating the region from the rest of China. Foremost among these is the Gobi Desert, which halted the advance of Chinese agriculture into the northwest.

Other formidable barriers to transportation and communication include massive mountain ranges, boasting some of the world's highest mountain peaks. To the north and northwest are the Tarbagatay Mountains, straddling the current border between Kazakstan and China. Several passes through these mountains have been used for centuries, providing avenues of access for Kazaks and other nomadic peoples of the Kazak and Jungarian (Dzungarian) steppes. Along the northeastern border, between Xinjiang and neighboring Mongolia, the Altay Mountains offer a similar barrier, permeable only to the hardiest of Mongol and Kazak nomads.

Equally impressive ranges rise in the south: The Altun Shan separate southeast Xinjiang from Qinghai, and the towering Kunlun separate it from Tibet, just to the south. In the southwestern corner, a knot of mountain ranges intersect: the Karakorum, the Hindu Kush, and the Pamirs, which together have limited human passage from the Far East into South Asia and present-day Afghanistan and Tajikistan.

In the west, the Tian Shan range arises in the northern part of neighboring Kyrgyzstan and enters Xinjiang just north of Kashgar. This massive range dominates the center of the region, varying from 250 to 300 kilometers wide and 1,700 kilometers in length. Its many valleys and streams provide hundreds of acres of pasturage to nomad flocks. It is also China's largest glacier area, with 6,890 glaciers covering some 7,790 square kilometers.[1] These glaciers are Xinjiang's greatest water source, supplying waters for the irrigation system used in the oases of the south and also feeding some of the region's huge natural lakes. The largest of these is Lake Bosten, which covers 980 square kilometers south of the Tian Shan in the Yanqi Basin. It is China's largest inland body of freshwater. Also important is Lake Ulungur, which lies to the north of the Tian Shan and covers 800 square kilometers. Both lakes are fed by the Tian Shan's snows and melting glaciers.

Geographically, the Xinjiang-Uyghur Autonomous Region can be divided into three distinct areas: the north, with its abundance of mountain pasturage and greater rainfall, which has been the province of nomadic peoples; the Tian Shan range, which also has afforded nomads pasturage, even while making possible oasis agriculture; and the much larger, more arid south, which is the home of over 80 percent of the sedentary Uyghur population. Although the south has not been the province of the Kazaks, it is intimately connected to their history. This part of Xinjiang is known as the Tarim Basin, the center of which is the Takla Makan Desert. The basin is the largest of its kind in the world, covering approximately 45 percent of the autonomous region. The desert at its center covers some 370,000 kilometers.[2] Circling the basin are oasis towns like Korla in the southern foothills of the Tian Shan, Aksu further west, Yarkand and Kashgar in the southwest corner, and Khotan (Hotan) and Keriya (Yutian) in the south and southeast. The easternmost loop of the circle is the former site of Lop Nor, once a great salt lake surrounded by marsh and reeds and fed by the Tarim River, China's longest inland river at over 1,000 kilometers. Today Lop Nor is gone, and only a dry lake bed remains; the waters of the Tarim have been diverted to new agricultural settlements all along its route since the 1950s, permanently transforming the northern rim of the Tarim Basin.

The Lop Nor area has been further degraded as a consequence of its being used by China's nuclear testing facility, located in the desert wastes of the eastern Tarim Basin. The Kazaks as well as other Xinjiang residents have repeatedly protested against testing there, adding to tensions in the region in the 1990s.

Xinjiang's dramatic and varied topography has been one reason for its relative underdevelopment. But a further factor in this has been its climate. Although the region is located in temperate latitudes—equivalent to southern Europe—the presence of encircling deserts and mountains, plus isolation from any large body of water, results in a wide range of temperatures and in an overall, marked degree of aridity. The Turpan Basin, in eastern Xinjiang, has recorded temperatures at over 47.8° Celsius, while Fuyun (Koktogay) in the Altay Mountains, has had lows of −50.8° Celsius. While those temperatures constitute extremes, even the average winter temperatures in northern Xinjiang are cold: In January they range from −13 to −30° Celsius. (The summer temperatures are more peasant, ranging in July from 18 to 27° Celsius.) The southern cities enjoy milder winters with a mean annual temperature of 10 to 20° Celsius.

Precipitation varies in the extreme across the region. While northern mountain areas receive up to 750 millimeters of rainfall annually, the Tarim Basin receives less than 100–200 millimeters a year at the edges and less than 10 millimeters a year at its center.[3] Despite its aridity, however, the area produces an abundance of food through extensive irrigation. Uyghur farmers rely on melting snow in the spring to feed rivers and streams, which in turn provide water for irrigation. Historically, this supply has been more than adequate to enable widespread intensive cultivation on the Tarim oases. In areas of extreme heat, like the Turpan Basin, local farmers rely on the *karez,* an underground system of wells and irrigation channels, to tap the abundant mountain waters. As a result, the oases of Hami (Komul) and Turpan have produced exquisite fruits as well as cereal grains for many centuries. In more recent years, cotton has become an important cash crop in irrigated areas.

Crops vary from north to south in accordance with climate and the availability of water. In Yarkand, for instance, the main crop in 1958 was corn, planted and thriving on about 40 percent of the land. Wheat and, as mentioned above, cotton have both increased in importance, along with flax and rice. In the relatively newly cultivated fields of the Altay, wheat is sowed in spring, along with some oats, barley, flax, and corn. Legumes and industrial crops are gaining in importance, along with sorghum and sugar beets.[4]

Some of the best soil in Xinjiang is in the north, especially along the Manas, Irtish, and Ulungur rivers in the north. All of these areas were nomad pasture lands; today they are sites for state farms established by the Production Construction Corp (hereafter PCC), a branch of the People's Liberation Army (PLA). The PCC has been effective in reclaiming land in the southern part of Xinjiang along the Tarim River, another area of agricultural development since 1949.

As suggested by its topography, Xinjiang is one of the great reservoirs of natural resources for China. Beneath the deserts of the Tarim Basin lie China's greatest oil reserves. Japanese and European companies now compete with Chinese enterprises for rights to develop these reserves, which constitute an extraordinary potential source of wealth for the state. The region's most developed oil field is at Karamay, north and west of the regional capital, Urumqi. Likewise, the rich mineral deposits of northern Xinjiang have been exploited for hundreds of years, yielding tin, copper, silver, and gold. The region also has abundant coal, uranium, and molybdenum.

Xinjiang's position on one of the world's once-great trade routes has historically brought other forms of wealth. Traders dealing in Chinese luxury goods were an important part of the economy; and services for traders—caravanserai, pack animals, local guides, and supplies—provided further sources of income for the oasis populations. The disruption of these important trade arteries in the fifteenth and sixteenth centuries meant a decrease in an important economic activity for many of the oasis towns; the development of sea routes to Asia further reduced the importance of the caravan trade, although it did not end it. However, despite the decline in trade, Xinjiang's oasis towns remained agricultural and trading centers, where local wares were offered in the markets alongside goods from neighboring states. The larger towns also served as centers of learning and religious activity. The urban areas thus assumed important economic and cultural roles, which evolved through many centuries of contact with surrounding states and empires. Though European explorers "discovered" the region once more in the late nineteenth century and reported a backward, remote and isolated land, this land, from an East Turkestani viewpoint, was at the very center of the Eurasian world.

While isolated from Europe by vast distances, Xinjiang was not isolated from the Islamic tradition of the Middle East, nor was it isolated from the influence of East Asia. By the twentieth century, religious and political elites in major towns and cities were already aware of pan-Turkic and pan-Islamic movements originating in the Middle East. The revolutions in China and Russia furthered local knowledge of nationalism, communism, and democracy—the latter as embodied in the new republics that sprouted all around the region in the first two decades of the new century. Both the sedentary and nomadic populations were increasingly influenced by these new ideas, flowing from both the east and the west.

The Peoples of Xinjiang: Their Distribution and History

Xinjiang is the home of the vast majority of China's Turkic-speaking Muslims as well as less numerous non-Han Chinese peoples that today are officially recognized as national minorities in the PRC. The follow-

Table 1.1

Populations of Contemporary Nationalities in Xinjiang

Nationality	1953	1982	1990
Uyghur	3,640,125	5,949,655	7,194,675
Han	300,000	5,286,532	5,695,626
Kazak	594,500	903,335	1,106,989
Hui	200,000	681,527	570,789
Kirghiz	70,000	112,973	139,781
Mongol	59,000	117,460	137,740
Xibo (Sibo)	13,600	27,364	33,082
Russian	13,000	2,662	8,082
Tajik	14,000	24,684	33,512
Uzbek	13,600	12,433	14,456
Tatar	6,900	4,106	4,821
Manchu	1,000	9,137	18,403
Tahur (Daur)	2,000	5,398	4,370
Others	—	54,333	81,686

Source: The 1953 and 1982 are from Linda Benson and Ingvar Svanberg, eds., Kazaks of China (1988), 35–36. The 1990 figures are from FBIS-CHI–90–250. December 28, 1990, 54.

ing sections briefly introduce the most historically important non-Kazak groups living in contemporary Xinjiang, all of whom have shared and shaped the modern history of China's Kazaks.

Uyghurs

Throughout the twentieth century, the single most numerous ethnic group in Xinjiang has been the Uyghur people, whose population was over 8 million in 1996. Because this group has been the dominant majority in Xinjiang historically, it is important to establish clearly both their identity and their relationship to the Kazaks.

The name "Uyghur" first appeared in the eighth century A.D., designating a people who ruled an ancient Turkic state founded in Mongolia. Modern Chinese historiography portrays the modern Uyghurs as the direct descendants of this ancient Uyghur kingdom, although not all historians agree on the extent of this ancient connection. The name "Uyghur" itself disappeared several hundred years ago, being revived only in the twentieth century. Unresolved issues of interpretation of the Uyhgur past, however, have not been an impediment to the development of a strong national consciousness among the people today known as the Uyghurs, who have come to constitute a single, coherent ethnic group with a clear sense of national identity.[5] The first Uyghur empire was founded in 744 A.D. by Qutlug Bilga (Kuli Peilo), and was based at Karakorum, in Mongolia. At that time, the neighboring Tang dynasty (618–906) was suffering from internal divisions in the court and military, which led to the An Lushan Rebellion in 755. The Tang emperor asked for Uyghur assistance in the struggle, and Uyghur intervention turned the tide in the court's favor. For their help in crushing the rebels, the Uyghur ruler was given a Chinese princess as his wife, the first of three such brides granted to Uyghur rulers between 762 and 840. The Tang debt to the Uyghurs resulted in increased trade between the two kingdoms, and Uyghur horses were traded for Chinese silk—often to the disadvantage of the Chinese. Nothing, however, could be done to redress Chinese traders' complaints about overpriced, poor quality mounts delivered to China, not as long as the Tang believed it might need Uyghur assistance.

During the rebellion, Uyghurs in the Tang capital of Changan (Xian) were introduced to the Manichaean religion, probably around 762. The Uyghur *khagan,* their ruler, was converted to the new faith, later imposing it upon his people as a state religion. In 768, a Manichaean temple was erected on the banks of the Orkhon River, in contemporary central Mongolia; and by the ninth century the religion was well entrenched.

Uyghur power on the steppe began to decline in the middle of the ninth century, as a result of court intrigue over the issue of succession. A series of natural calamities in 839 further weakened the power of the Uyghur elite. In 840, the capital of Karakorum was attacked, and in subsequent battles the ruling clan was defeated by a Kirghiz chieftain—who was at the head of 100,000 men, according to ancient Chinese sources. They stormed the capital and beheaded the Uyghur ruler. Consequently, "the Uyghurs scattered and fled all over the barbarian territory."[6]

While some remnants of the ancient Uyghurs joined other Turkic groups in what is now Mongolia, others fled to present-day Xinjiang, establishing centers at Kocho, Beshbalik, and, later, at Kuqa. Here they modified their nomadic lifestyle and began to assume the characteristics of a sedentary oasis population. In 840 A.D., the year of the Uyghur arrival, Xinjiang was already populated by an Indo-European people who had established themselves centuries earlier in settlements on the banks of the Tarim River. These small towns served the traders on what came to be called the Silk Road, along which a variety of goods moved between China and the great trading cities of the West. Initially under the rule of their own kings, the Indo-Europeans had been forced by 635 to accept Chinese suzerainty. When the Uyghurs arrived, the Indo-Europeans remained nominally under Chinese rule. As Chinese dynastic fortunes waned, however, the Uyghurs spread their domains through the various oasis settlements, creating an empire that eventually stretched from Turpan in the east to Kuqa in the west by 1017 A.D.

During the period between the eleventh and thirteenth centuries, Uyghur society showed a remarkable religious tolerance, allowing Nestorian Christianity to flourish, along with Zoroastrianism and Buddhism. Barthold, the great historian of Central Asian history, has commented that among the Uyghurs were representatives of all major religious faiths except Judaism. Possibly this tolerance contributed to the spread of Uyghur cultural influence, which came to dominate not only the northern oases, but also the towns and cities of the Tarim basin.

In 1211, the Uyghur ruler Barchuq submitted to Chinggis Khan, whose troops entered the area in the early thirteenth century. The Great Khan gave his daughter Al-Altun to Barchuq in marriage. As a further mark of favor, Chinggis Khan decreed that his sons be taught by Uyghur tutors and that Mongol nobility be taught to write in the Uyghur script, which is the basis of the modern script of Mongolia. The Uyghurs themselves abandoned this ancient form for the Arabic script after their conversion to Islam. Following the death of Chinggis Khan, the Mongol domains were divided; control over the Uyghur lands declined, allowing local Uyghur rulers once more to rule the oases.

During the eleventh century, Islam extended its influence throughout the Kashgar area. This new religion gradually spread among the Uyghurs, moving north and east from the southern oases until, by the sixteenth century, the population as far east as Komul (Hami) was converted. The new religion provided a new ethnonym, "Mohammedan," which was used by the Chinese as a general name for the inhabitants of the northwest. Rulers of the oasis city-states honored Islam, some claiming descent from the family of the Prophet and/or from the heirs of Chinggis Khan to underpin their claims to power. No single state emerged, however, until the nineteenth century.

In 1644, the Qing dynasty (1644–1912) arose in China, bringing the Manchu people to the throne. By the eighteenth century this powerful foreign dynasty began the conquest of what was then called the Western Regions. By 1759 the whole of the Xinjiang region was under Qing control. As part of Manchu policy, some 10,000 Uyghur families from the Tarim Basin were moved to the Ili area in order to provide crops and a labor force for the Manchu garrison stationed there. This group of Uyghurs came to be known as the Taranchi, meaning "tillers of the soil," a name no longer used today.

By the time of the Qing conquests, the population of Xinjiang reflected centuries of intermingling among the many peoples who had variously inhabited or conquered and dominated the region. The original Persian-speaking Indo-Europeans of the south, the Mongol invaders from the east and north, and the representatives of the Chinese empire had all left their mark, culturally and physically, on the local population. The name "Uyghur" virtually disappeared under the Qing. The local population was commonly referred to as Mohammedan or Turki, the latter being a name still used in the 1940s to describe the Uyghurs. Locally, people identified themselves by referring to their religion—calling themselves Mohammedan, for example—or, depending on the situation, simply by using the name of their native town. A man from Kashgar was referred to as a Kashgarlik and a man from Khotan as a Khotanlik, and so on.

In the nineteenth century, the region's Muslim population repeatedly rose against their Qing rulers. They were joined by the Hui (the Chinese Muslims) in opposing what was considered an oppressive, infidel regime, staging rebellions in 1815, 1825, 1830, 1847, and 1857. By the 1860s much of northwestern China had risen in rebellion against the Qing, paving the way for the insurrection of Yakub Beg. From his position under the Khan as a governor of the Kokand Khanate, Yakub Beg had risen to become the military leader of forces in Kashgar, whence the Khan had sent him in 1865. By 1870 Yakub Beg controlled all of southern Xinjiang and part of the north. Although the new ruler was a native of Central Asia and a Muslim, he was not Uyghur. His conservative Islamic rule became highly unpopular; furthermore, according to a Russian observer of the day, most peasants were able to keep only one-fourth to one-half of their produce, the rest being taken in taxes. This oppressive rate of taxation was one reason why the local population reportedly rejoiced when Qing armies entered the area, crushing the rebellion in 1876. Yakub Beg himself died in 1877, supposedly by his own hand. The region once more came under the influence of China, represented by victorious General Zuo Zongtang, who restored order and firmly reestablished Chinese control in Xinjiang.[7] In 1884, the Qing court made the region a province and gave it the name of Xinjiang ("New Dominion").

The Chinese revolution of 1911 did not end Chinese control of Xinjiang. Instead, the area passed into the hands of a series of warlords, leading to a rebellion against Chinese rule in 1931 that began in Hami and then spread into the south. In 1933 Muslim leaders established the East Turkestan Republic at Kashgar, one of the leaders of which was Khodja Niaz, of a prominent Muslim family. In response, troops of the province's most capable military leader, Sheng Shicai— allied alternately with White Russian and, briefly, with Soviet forces— suppressed the republic, executing some leaders and driving others into exile. Victorious, Sheng established himself as the local warlord, dominating the province until his departure in 1944. The East Turkestan Republic would be revived in that year.

Prior to Sheng's takeover, the local population was most commonly called the *Chantou* by the Chinese while nomads and Russians called them *Sart*. It was under the rule of Sheng Shicai that the name "Uyghur" was reintroduced into the region. In doing so, Sheng deferred to his Soviet mentors and advisors, who had revived the name reportedly at the request of Uyghurs living in the USSR. At a meeting in Tashkent in 1921, this group had formally requested that "Uyghur" be used as their proper national identification, and the Soviet government had acquiesced in their request. In 1926 the Soviet census listed Uyghurs as one of its Central Asian peoples.

Initially, Sheng fostered a new sense of Uyghur identity by encouraging cultural activities for each of the region's ethnic groups. As in the USSR, this policy was one means by which to divide the local Muslim population by positing separate identities and nurturing competitive rather than cooperative relations. Muslim intellectuals continued to prefer being designated as Turki or East Turkestani, and a number of groups sought to counter government efforts to establish separate identities for the Muslim Turkic peoples in the region. When the East Turkestan Republic was founded in 1944 by a coalition of Uyghurs, Kazaks, and other local ethnic groups, Muslim and Turki remained the most common identifications for the local population.

After 1949, guided by Soviet advice, the PRC continued the use of the name "Uyghur," following what was originally a Nationalist policy. The name was used in all official documents, in the press, and on all official occasions. By the end of the century, the name was considered the correct and appropriate designation for the majority of the sedentary oases population.

As in the past, Uyghurs today are Sunni Muslims, of the Hanafi juridical school. Traditionally oasis peasants, merchants, and traders, they are now also employed in the many new enterprises in rapidly developing Xinjiang. Handicrafts reflective of the Uyghur past continue to be produced, both for the local and the tourist market, the most famous products being carpets, traditional musical instruments, and metalwork.

The Uyghur language is closely related to Uzbek and was traditionally written in the Arabic script. When the printing of literary works and newspapers expanded in the region, the Taranchi dialect, also written in Arabic, was made the standard written form, following Soviet practice; it remains the standard form today. However, in southern Xinjiang, where the majority of the Uyghurs live, a number of local dialects continue to be spoken.

The Uyghurs were the most numerous single group in Xinjiang for centuries, comprising 75–80 percent of Xinjiang's population before 1949; however, by the 1990s they were less than half. This relative decrease has resulted mainly from the influx of Han Chinese settlers, who account today for approximately 40 percent of the region's population.

Han Chinese

Prior to the establishment of the PRC, the Han Chinese were one of the least numerous groups in Xinjiang. Under the last dynasty and in the republican era (1912–1949), no attempt was made to integrate the area fully into the Chinese political system, and few Chinese had any interest in moving to what was viewed as an uncivilized outpost.

During the Qing dynasty, the imperial court in Beijing sought to encourage Chinese settlers to emigrate into what is now Xinjiang by issuing an edict in 1776 that allowed a subsidy to be paid to all Han Chinese who settled in the northwest.[8] But the distant region was climatically and topographically unsuited to Chinese agriculture, and even the promise of financial assistance did not attract many settlers.

In the eighteenth century, a small number of traders and peasants made their way to Xinjiang, primarily to service the garrisons stationed there and to trade for local produce. Other Chinese were exiles—errant officials or criminals banished by the Qing court.

For Chinese who lived in Xinjiang prior to the twentieth century, life was often difficult and, in times of rebellion, extremely dangerous. During the rebellion of northwest Muslims and the struggle with Yakub Beg in the middle of the nineteenth century, some 40,000 Chinese died in Xinjiang.[9]

The Manchu government sent the Han Chinese general Zuo Zongtang to put down the rebellions and reestablish Qing control. General Zuo moved into the northwest slowly, using the *tuntian* system of having the soldiers stop to grow their own food in military settlements en route. As the army moved slowly west, traders and merchants followed in its wake. Once the rebellion was successfully quelled and order restored, some of the merchants and traders as well as a number of soldiers chose to settle in the region, availing themselves of the rich natural resources and many opportunities to do business.[10]

Many of the Chinese who remained were from Zuo's home province of Hunan. Others came from Yunnan, Gansu, and Manchuria. So many settlers from the coastal city of Tianjin moved into the Ili area that they were said to form their own complete community.[11] Chinese residents maintained separate communities within the cities of Xinjiang, a practice that continued at the end of the twentieth century.

After the founding of the new republic in 1912, there were again a few attempts to encourage Chinese to move to Xinjiang. Small numbers were lured to the region by promises of assistance, particularly from hard-hit famine areas such as Hunan and Gansu. However, most of these settlers moved no further west than the oasis of Hami, just at the western edge of the Gobi Desert. Despite government efforts, the Han population remained around 5 percent.

In the 1940s the first major Han Chinese influx took place: This time the new arrivals were neither exiles nor settlers, but were Chinese military units sent to suppress the 1944 Ili rebellion based in Yining (Gulja) and to secure Nationalist control over the other districts in the region. By 1946, there were an estimated 90,000 Han Chinese troops in Xinjiang, troops that placed a major economic burden on the local population. When the region was incorporated into the PRC in 1949, the surrendered Nationalist troops remained, incorporated into the new paramilitary

PCC, which began massive land reclamation projects in the region in the 1950s. By 1956, the PCC operated thirty-nine of the region's forty-four state farms and was poised to move into new enterprises.

In the late 1950s, the central government sent some 100,000 Han settlers to the area; and these were followed in the early 1960s by thousands more, swelling the Chinese population, particularly in the northern part of the region. A majority of the new arrivals were from Shanghai and coastal cities; Shanghai alone sent some 100,000 youngsters to work in the PCC. While some of this group eventually returned to Shanghai, roughly half remained as permanent settlers.[12]

The increase in the number of Han Chinese in Xinjiang constitutes one of the most dramatic demographic shifts in twentieth-century China. From being only approximately 5 percent of the population before 1949, by the 1990s they constituted nearly 40 percent of the total. Han Chinese influence has never been this pervasive in all of the region's previous recorded history, and the ramifications of this shift in the ethnic composition is a major challenge to minorities like the Kazaks.

Xinjiang's Minorities

The Uyghurs, Han Chinese, and Kazaks are the three most numerous nationalities in Xinjiang today. According to the 1990 census, the region is now also home to members of forty-seven different nationalities, some represented by only a handful of recent settlers.[13] In addition to these relative newcomers, the region remains the home of groups that have been there for the last two centuries, most of whom have substantial populations. Nationalities with a population between 100,000 and 1 million include the Hui, or Chinese Muslims; the Kirghiz, and the Mongols. Other groups sharing a long history with the Kazaks include the Xibo, Manchu, Russian, Tajik, Uzbek, and Tatar peoples, each of which is introduced briefly below.

The Hui

The Hui are Chinese-speaking Muslims who live in towns scattered throughout Xinjiang. In the former USSR, they were known as Dungans, which is the name still used for them by Kazaks. In China, their total 1990 population was 8,602,978; in the same year, 570,789 lived in Xinjiang.

The origins of the Hui are said to date from the seventh century, when Muslim traders first arrived in China. At the time of the Mongols' Yuan dynasty, traders from the Middle East were allowed to live in China; records from that period refer to these men and their Chinese families as Hui Hui. Many of the descendants of these marriages became soldiers in the service of the Chinese, beginning a military tradition that has lasted down through the centuries. Dispersed throughout China, many became fully sinified, with only their refusal to eat pork and their attendance at mosque separating them from other Chinese.[14] As coreligionists, they have joined the Uyghurs and Kazaks against the Chinese in Xinjiang, allying with these larger groups in the Qing period and again during the republican era.

Xinjiang's Hui are Sunni Muslims, like the Turkic-speaking Muslims of the region. Unlike them, however, they belong to the Shafi juridical school, rather than to the Hanafi. Hui mosques also differ from those of the Turkic peoples, being built mainly in the Chinese architectural style. In 1990, 23 percent of the region's Hui lived in the largest cities; another 50 percent lived in the Ili-Kazak and Changji Hui Autonomous Prefectures.

Kirghiz (Kyrghyz)

Xinjiang's Kirghiz population was 139,781 in 1990, according to the census of that year. They are an extension of the Kirghiz people who, like the Soviet Kazaks, found themselves possessed of an independent republic upon the abrupt collapse of the USSR in 1991. Like the Kazaks, they are traditionally pastoral nomads, grazing their herds and flocks in mountainous areas of southern Xinjiang and in the Ili River valley. After 1949, the PRC provided an autonomous prefecture for them, the Kizilsu-Kirghiz Autonomous Prefecture in southern Xinjiang, which abuts Tajikistan and Kyrgyzstan, the latter being the preferred spelling in the new republic. They are Sunni Muslims of the Hanafi school, like the Uyghurs and Kazaks.

Mongols

According to the 1990 census, Xinjiang is home to 137,740 Mongols, most of whom live in the northern third of the region. Several autonomous areas have been created for them since 1949, including the

Bortala- and Bayingolin-Mongol Autonomous Prefectures and the Hoboksar (Koluk Saur) Mongol Autonomous County. In both the Mongolian prefectures, Mongols are a minority: As of 1990, in Bortala, there were 23,467 Mongols out of a total population of 328,005; and in Bayangol, there were 41,157 out of 839,162. Han Chinese constitute the largest single nationality in both areas.[15] Mainly the descendants of Oirat or Torgut Mongols, the majority speak a western Mongolian language. A small number of Chakhar Mongols, originally from the area of Inner Mongolia, arrived during the Qing period; they speak a southern Mongolian language. The region also has a small number of Uriangkhai Mongols, originally from the Tanu Tuva area, directly north of Xinjiang. Although their vocabulary is dominated by Mongolian borrowings, they are nonetheless regarded as Turkic-speaking by scholars. Little is known about their status in contemporary Xinjiang, but they are still identified as Mongols rather than as a Turkic people.

The Daur minority is another Mongolian-speaking group, most of whom live near the town of Tacheng (Qochek), near the Kazakstan border. Until the early 1950s, they were called Solon in official records, a name dating from the Qing dynasty, when the Manchu government sent Solons from Manchuria to Xinjiang as military settlers. It is said that the descendants of the Solons themselves requested that they be renamed as Daurs in 1954. According to Chinese census figures, their population has varied from only 2,000 in 1953 to 5,398 in 1982 and down to 4,370 in 1990.[16] In 1991, their population in Xinjiang rose again to 6,383; although there is no autonomous jurisdiction for them, the majority (4,491) live in the Tacheng district, many on the Gurbansher-Daur commune; another 439 live in the neighboring Ili district.[17] Relatively little information is available on this small group, but the government provides some cultural support, recently publishing a Daur-Kazak-Han dictionary.

Another Mongolian-speaking group are the Dongxiang, recent immigrants from neighboring Gansu province. In the 1950s, there were only a few Dongxiang families living in Xinjiang, but by 1958 some 30,000 had settled in the city of Yining, capital of the Ili-Kazak Autonomous Prefecture.[18] By 1982 they numbered 40,318 (out of total for all of China of 279,397). In contrast to other Mongolian-speaking groups in Xinjiang, who are Lama Buddhists, the Dongxiang are Sunni Muslims.

Xibo and Manchu

All the minority groups introduced above speak Turkic languages or Mongolian languages belonging to the Altaic family. A third branch of the family represented in Xinjiang is the Manchu-Tungus group. The most numerous minority in this language category are the Xibo (Sibo), Manchu-speaking inhabitants of the Ili River valley, west of Yining. They arrived as part of the Manchu garrisons assigned to the area in the eighteenth century. By 1900, they numbered about 25,000, living in seven villages organized according to the Manchu banner system.[19] As of 1990, 27,315 out of a total of 33,082 Xibo in Xinjiang lived in the Ili-Kazak Autonomous Prefecture, of which the Qapqal-Xibo Autonomous County is a part. The next largest concentration of Xibo is in Urumqi, which had a Xibo population of 2,693 in 1990.[20] Since the early 1980s there has been a literary revival among Manchu speakers like the Xibo, resulting in numerous books being published in the traditional Manchu script.

The next largest Manchu-Tungus group is the Manchu minority itself. In the early 1950s, few people evidently felt comfortable in identifying themselves as Manchus; but as the benefits of identification with a specific minority nationality emerged, the number of Manchus in China jumped dramatically, from 4.3 million in 1982 to 9.8 million in 1990. A similar phenomenon occurred in Xinjiang: The 1982 census listed 9,137 Manchus, but by 1990 the number was 18,403—more than double the 1982 level. Interest in the study of Manchu language and literature has increased; as noted above, publishing in the traditional Manchu script was revived in the 1980s, although the number of Manchus who actually read—or speak—their own language is unknown.

Another Manchu-speaking group mentioned in the 1953 Chinese census are the Solons, a name that disappeared after 1954, as previously explained in connection with the Daurs. This group not only included the Daurs, but also a group that referred to themselves as Evenki. According to early twentieth-century sources, a Manchu-speaking people in western Xinjiang identified themselves as Evenki but were more commonly referred to as Solons, their Manchu banner name. In 1962, twenty Evenki were reportedly living in the same area. They were identified as being Ongkor-Evenks, descendants of Qing bannermen brought to the area in the 1760s, remaining in the Tacheng area.[21] Both these names—Solon and Evenki—have disappeared from

Chinese census figures, and it is not known whether any individuals today regard themselves as members of either group. As these were very small communities, most likely they have been assimilated into larger groups such as the Manchu-speaking Xibo.

In the Altay area there is also another small ethnic group, the so-called Kokmonchaq, said to speak a mixed Kazak-Mongol-Solon vernacular.[22] According to linguist Geng Shimin, there is also a small community of 2,000 Tuvins in the Altay area, and it seems likely that these are actually the same as the Kokmonchaq.[23]

Russians

For at least a hundred years, Russians have also constituted a minority population in Xinjiang. After the Bolshevik Revolution, hundreds of so-called Whites—those opposed to the "Reds," or Bolsheviks—retreated into Xinjiang. Some of these were repatriated by the local governor in the 1920s, while others were able to move on to the Chinese coast. Those who remained in the northwest made their living in a variety of ways, including farming or trading; several thousand Russian men also enlisted in the local military. By 1949, the province had 19,500 ethnic Russians. Their numbers steadily decreased, and by 1982 only 2,662 remained. Between 1982 and 1990, however, numbers fluctuated; in the 1990 census, the number of Russians was up to 8,082, suggesting that, like the Manchus, individuals who had not previously registered as Russian were now choosing to do so. As with other smaller minorities, relatively little information is available about the present circumstances of China's Russians. The three largest concentrations of Russians live in Urumqi (2,180), Tacheng (2,762), and the Ili area (1,058).[24]

Tajiks

As a Persian-speaking minority, the Tajiks of Xinjiang represent the Indo-European family of languages. They are inhabitants of the Pamirs, where the government established the Tashkurgan-Tajik Autonomous County, and their 1990 population of 33,512 was concentrated in the far southwest of the region, with small numbers scattered elsewhere through the westernmost counties of Xinjiang. Small groups of Tajiks also live around the towns of Guma, Yarkand, and Poskam.

Unlike other Muslims in the region, the Tajiks belong to the Ismaili sect of Shi'a Islam. The majority raise animals and cultivate those crops that do well at higher elevations, such as wheat and barley.

Uzbeks

In 1990, Xinjiang's Uzbek population was 14,456. The largest concentration of these Turkic Muslim people live in the Ili area, which in 1990 was home to 5,899 Uzbeks. Some 3,500 lived in the Kashgar area, and 1,300 lived in Urumqi. Smaller numbers are scattered throughout the region. As the Uzbek language is very close to Uyghur, Xinjiang's Uzbeks mix easily with the Uyghurs, and their children attend Uyghur schools in most areas. Since the independence of Uzbekistan, some have sought to emigrate and rejoin immediate family or other relatives. Uzbeks have joined the new cohort of traders who act as middlemen for the China–Central Asian trade. Mainly urban dwellers, Uzbeks in Xinjiang work as businessmen, craftsmen, and teachers.

Tatars

The Tatars of Xinjiang are Sunni Muslims, mostly of Kazan Tatar origin and who immigrated to Xinjiang from Russia at the end of the nineteenth century. They are one of the least numerous of the minorities surveyed here, and their overall population has remained under 5,000. A modest increase was recorded from 1982 to 1990, when the population rose from 4,106 to 4,821. The three largest concentrations are in the Changji-Hui Autonomous Prefecture, the Altay district, and the Ili area, each with about 1,000 Tatars. Although their numbers were never very large, a reminder of their contribution to the region's history can be found in Urumqi, where the Tatar Mosque still stands, not far from the University of Xinjiang.

Conclusion

The brief descriptions given above of some of Xinjiang's many minority peoples convey an image of great cultural and linguistic diversity. This multiethnic collage suggests a potential for endless conflict over resources, as well as over cultural and religious differences. However, while there has been some conflict, the region's size and varied topography have allowed many of these groups to fill specific geographical niches, with nomadic peoples like the Mongols, Kazaks, and Tajiks living in more mountainous areas—some of which are extremely isolated—and sedentary groups like the Uyghur, Uzbek, Tatar, and Russians sharing oasis and urban life in relative equanimity.

The sparseness of the population has been another factor in cultural accommodation in Xinjiang. It has only been since 1949 that the populations described above have had to contend with shrinking availability of land and water for animal herds and with the ecological demands of a new manufacturing and industrial sector in the economy. Reclamation of land for agriculture has facilitated a huge overall increase in population of the region, the majority of which is represented by the newly arrived Han Chinese. Cities have grown as never before, drawing both the Chinese and local minorities to the new urban environment. While ethnic strife historically has pitted Muslim peoples against the Chinese, ethnic relations are clearly entering a new phase as populations once isolated by miles of deserts and mountains now increasingly have access to one another.

The single most dramatic change is the arrival of millions of Han Chinese since the late 1950s, a fact of demographic life that none of the minorities can ignore. Though sharing the Muslim faith and a Turkic origin with several of Xinjiang's minority groups, the Kazaks will increasingly find that relations with the Han Chinese will be their most important intercultural interaction— outweighing both their differences and similarities with Xinjiang's other minority groups.

——— 2 ———
Kazaks in Central Eurasia and China to the Twentieth Century

Origins

The present-day Kazak people are an integral part of Central Eurasia's history—a history not yet fully explored and only partially recorded. The Kazaks' Turkic language links them to the great Turkic-Mongol-speaking confederations and empires that rose and fell over many centuries in ancient Central Eurasia. They are part of a Central Asian culture that includes ancient peoples such as the Saka, Wusun, Hun, and Yuezhi, who roamed with their herds and flocks over two thousand years ago. As these peoples disappear from written sources, successors to the same lands emerge—known to us as the Toba, Turk, Uyghur, and Karluk—peoples who lived in the third to eighth centuries A.D. Until the earliest forms of written Turkish appeared in the eighth century A.D., Central Eurasian history was recorded only intermittently by neighboring literate, settled peoples to both the east and the west. As representatives of agricultural empires, these chroniclers regarded the largely nomadic Central Eurasians as uncivilized and dangerous, possessed of many animals but of no fixed abode, practicing many "primitive and quaint" rites but having no government. Alternately scorning and fearing the nomads, the accounts that have come down to us over the centuries give only partial clues to the reality of steppe life in ancient times. Reconstructing any kind of coherent picture of Central Asian peoples prior to the eighth century on the basis of such accounts remains a difficult business, open to a broad range of interpretations.

The still-limited findings of archaeologists have begun to influence recent historical writing about the region, but only modestly. Studies such as Maenchen-Helfen's *World of the Huns* (1973) and Sinor's *Cambridge History of Inner Asia* (1990) reflect application of archaeological discoveries, as does recent work in Russian and European languages.[1] Chinese scholars are also utilizing such findings to inform new studies of peoples like the Kazaks, although the political agendas behind some of these writings are not only distracting but at times misleading.[2]

Work by both archaeologists and the relatively small number of historians interested in Central Eurasian history over the past century and a half still allows only tentative conclusions on the Kazaks' origins. As Olcott observes in her 1987 study of Kazaks in the USSR, claims for a single Kazak people inhabiting the vast Kazak steppe from earliest times to the present remain unverifiable.[3]

Who, then, are the Kazaks? First, as noted above, they are part of the great Turkic-Mongol confederations whose earliest known origins are on lands extending from present-day central Mongolia to the Altay Mountains of northwestern China. Measured by stone implements and other artifacts, human habitation of the Altay has been traced through both the Paleolithic and Neolithic periods, and several successive cultures are now generally accepted as having occupied this region in the second millennium B.C. By the time the earliest written Turkic language appears in the eighth century A.D., Turkic and Mongol peoples dominated the northern steppes, providing a verifiable link between Turkic peoples of the past and those of the present day.

Second, the Kazaks have exhibited the traditional Central Eurasian pattern of nomadism shared by all the great confederations, from Saka to Mongol, that rose on the steppes. As is true of other great Central Eurasian peoples of today—the Uyghur, Uzbek, Kirghiz, Turkmen, and Mongols—Kazak socioeconomic organization derived from pastoral nomadism, as do many Kazak cultural traits, which reflect the requirements of a nomadic lifestyle.

Like other Central Eurasian peoples, the Kazaks' steppe heritage has included a form of social organization that began with the clan, expanded to the tribe, and culminated in the confederation. Vestiges of shamanism remained despite the Kazaks' adherence to Islam, as was true for other Central Eurasians into the twentieth century.[4] As discussed below, birth, marriage, and burial rites among the Kazaks have also continued to reflect the greater Turkic steppe traditions.

Although these broad categories of Turkic, Islamic, and nomadic distinguish Central Eurasians from the settled agriculturists of the empires that rose in Europe, the Middle East, and Asia, the differentiation of specific Central Eurasian peoples today lies in the confederations that represented the most complex form of political organization on the steppe prior to the nineteenth century. Although these confederations were usually organized for specific goals and were largely temporary steppe phenomena, they provided a basis for cohesion in the early modern period from which emerged most of the modern Central Eurasian peoples.

The Kazaks are one of several such peoples whose origins begin with a confederation. Historically, the most powerful confederation to emerge on the steppes was that of the Mongols under Chinggis Khan, whose confederated alliance included both Mongol and Turkic-speaking clans. Among the latter were the Uyghurs of Turpan and Beshbalik who joined voluntarily. Other Turkic-speaking peoples were forced to join after defeat on the battlefield. During the course of the thirteenth century Mongol conquests, no people under the name of Kazak appear among the khan's subjects. But by the sixteenth century the Kazaks, under their own leader or khan, emerged as one of the heirs to the former Mongol empire.

Before turning to this aspect of the Kazaks' origins, let us look briefly at recent Chinese sources that seek to trace a clear line of descent for the Kazaks from ancient times to the present. Doing so allows us to examine some of the problems inherent in such an enterprise and to understand why the issue of ethnic origin—for the Kazaks as well as for other contemporary peoples of northwestern China—remains problematic.

Beginning in the 1980s, books on Kazak history began appearing in China that emphasized the long and close ties between the Kazaks, now officially a national minority of the Chinese communist state, and the Han Chinese. As was the case for virtually all other minorities in China,[5] Chinese accounts of the Kazaks' origins link present-day Kazaks to ancient Central Eurasian peoples whose roots are firmly planted in the territory of the contemporary Chinese state. For scholars of Kazak history in China, this has meant a search to connect present-day Kazaks to a specific, historically identifiable people whose earliest traceable origins are clearly Chinese. Thus far, the group so designated by Chinese researchers is the Wusun, who first appear in Chinese records as living in the area of Dunhuang, an ancient town on the old Silk Road, with a respectably ancient history of some 2,500 years. The

Wusun people moved west, to the Ili River valley, around the third century B.C. Here they merged with the Saka, known in Chinese records as the Saizhong. The Wusun-Saka tribes of this area include the Jersak, Bessak, Bersak, and Kazsak, the name of the latter tribe providing a linguistic link to the Kazaks. While these Wusun-Saka tribes are not presented as the only source of the modern Kazak people, they are considered by Chinese historians to be one of the most important elements of the later modern nation.[6]

The presence of thousands of Kazaks in the Ili Valley today and the ancient presence there of the Wusun tribe of Kazsak are events separated by two millennia. A succession of peoples and rulers claimed this land, as periods of war and devastation, of peace and prosperity were all marked by migrations into and out of the region. Unrecorded by the peoples themselves, it fell to their literate Chinese neighbors—at a distance of over 1,000 miles to the east—to reconstruct what happened there as the centuries passed. Excellent record keepers, the authors of Chinese imperial histories described the Western Regions as being inhabited by numerous peoples. But imprecise and sometimes conflicting information makes it difficult to trace with certainty any direct lines of descent. Thus, while we know of Chinese attitudes toward these populations and have a record of Chinese interaction through a number of dynasties, the relationship of these groups to each other is difficult to assess, as is the line of descent from one group to another. It is only conjecture today that can link a specific tribe like the ancient Kazsak tribe of the Wusun confederation to a modern people.

This is not to say that the modern Kazaks have no traceable past. Indeed, as suggested earlier, the Kazaks are without doubt a part of a much larger picture that, though not clear in its specific detail, nonetheless allows us to place them within the broad framework of Turkic civilization in Central Eurasia. From early modern times, we have available a quantity of more reliable records, of both the Eastern and Western historiographical traditions, that help to identify an emerging Kazak nation in the fifteenth century, already building on the rich heritage of a shared Turkic past.

The Kazak Khanate

The origins of the Kazak confederation—not the people but the political organization out of which the modern identity was born—lay with the heirs of the great Chinggis Khan, who led the united Mongol and Turkic tribes in conquering the city-states and lands of Central Eurasia in the 1220s. After the death of the khan, the Mongol empire was divided among his heirs. Chinggis's grandson, Batu, became leader of a confederation of mainly Turkic tribes known as the White Horde. Their lands extended from northwest of the Black Sea to north of the Caspian and into the central part of present-day Kazakstan. The White Horde enjoyed an income derived from trade and taxation, and its leadership was handed down through brothers, according to Mongol practice. In 1428, leadership of this confederation was contested, and one of the candidates for the throne, Barak Khan, was assassinated by his rival, Abulkhair Khan (Abu'l Khayr). Fearing retribution, Barak Khan's two sons fled or were forced to flee in the 1450s. These two men, Janibek and Giray (Kirai, or Girei) led some 200,000 followers west, seeking refuge in what was then Western Mogholistan, which controlled lands between Issyk Kul and Kashgar. The Moghol khan, Esenburqa, granted them lands in the area of the river Chu.

Here the brothers and their supporters, with their flocks and herds, were able to thrive. They successfully protected themselves against the army of Abulkhair Khan in 1468, killing both the khan and his son in brutal fighting. According to traditional, oral genealogical accounts, Janibek's son, Kasim Khan, succeeded to the throne in 1511.[7]

Kasim Khan was responsible for extending Kazak control over nearby territories, and gained recognition as the leader of a powerful confederation that dominated not only steppe lands but also cities along the Syr Darya River. Members of this confederation became known as Kazak people, and by the time of Kasim Khan's death in 1523, the million-strong Kazak confederation provided a foundation for an increasingly cohesive people.

While this brief history is generally accepted as our most accurate account of the Kazaks' modern origins, explanations of the origins of the name itself vary widely. These range from mythic legends, to identifying ancient ancestors with similar-sounding names, to examining linguistic evidence. Kazaks in China often use the latter, seeing in the Turkish words *kaz* (goose) and *ak* (white), the true origin of their name. Their ancestor myth ascribes Kazak origins to a white goose of the steppes that turned into a princess and bore a male child, who became the first Kazak. Other accounts seem equally fanciful—some even less plausible. As with many other steppe names, from

"Cimmerian" to "Saka" and "Uyghur," the origin of "Kazak" remains a topic of conjecture and dispute. No one, however, disputes that by the middle of the sixteenth century, both the name and the confederation to which it referred were well established.

Ultimately, the great sedentary empires of Russia and China expanded into Kazak lands, seeking greater prestige and power as well as greater control over the often troublesome peripheries of their growing empires. As the Russian and Chinese empires expanded in a final, aggressive assertion of imperium in the eighteenth and nineteenth centuries, Kazak lands were enclosed and divided by new boundaries, signifying an end to millennia of nomad domination of Asia's vast "heartland."

Kazaks in Qing China (1644–1912)

Imperial China traditionally claimed jurisdiction over Central Asia, but in reality the Chinese were seldom able to control this region. In 751, during the Tang dynasty (618–906), a defeat of Chinese armies at the river Talas by Arabian forces marks the geographic extent of China's penetration into Central Asia; thereafter, the Chinese were only intermittently able to enforce control over the oasis cities of what is today the Xinjiang region. During the period of the Yuan (1276–1368), Mongols ruled both China and Central Asia. With the Yuan's defeat by the Chinese, a new dynastic power, the Ming (1368–1644), sought trade, not conquest, in the lands of Central Eurasia. Ming rulers received envoys from towns such as Hami and Turpan, through which trade continued between East and West. Other oases farther west were ruled by local elites, while those farthest from China's borders—Aksu and Kashgar—came under the control of Muslim rulers who were heir to the khanates of the Mongol period.

While the Ming brought peace to China and began a long, relatively stable period for the Chinese, the eastern portions of Central Eurasia (Eastern Turkestan) were sites of continued maneuverings for power by ambitious rulers seeking control over not only the steppes, but also wealthy trading centers throughout the region.

At the same time, to the northeast of the Chinese Ming state, yet another tribal confederation emerged, this time led by Tungus tribes and their closest Mongol neighbors. As the power of the Ming waned, emboldened by the Chinese court's disarray, the great leader Nurhaci led his clansmen and burgeoning Mongol allies in repeated incursions of Chinese territory. Nurhaci's heir, Abahai (Huang Taiji) renamed his people as the Manchu in 1636, and further consolidated and strengthened a Manchu-Mongol alliance through repeated marriages and battlefield victories. Having gained the services of disgruntled Ming generals, the Manchu-led confederation successfully invaded China in 1644, placing Nurhaci's heirs on the Throne of Heaven and naming their new dynasty the Qing (1644–1912).

Nurhaci's people had been nomads and hunters; but they had also established trading relations with China and had, in Nurhaci's day, already begun to follow the Chinese imperial model of rulership. Their capital city of Mukden, present-day Shenyang, was designed in imitation of the Chinese capital at Beijing; and successive generations of Manchu rulers adopted Chinese practices at court and in their new domains. Although these changes imply a sinification of the Qing court, the early Qing rulers enjoyed a different status in Mongolia and Central Asia than had their Chinese predecessors, and their alliances with the eastern Mongol tribes would provide a foundation for an empire far greater than that of the Ming.

Despite the Mongol alliance, however, the Qing empire was not free from troubles in its northern domains. In its first half century, the Qing dynasty was faced with the rising power of another great nomadic confederation, that of the Oyrat, the western Mongols.[8]

Under leadership of the assertive Jungar tribe, the western Mongols' confederation dominated Eastern Turkestan for over a hundred years. During the second half of the seventeenth century, under their leader Galdan Khan, the Jungars extended their influence from western Mongolia across a large portion of Central Asia, creating a powerful, independent nomadic state. The Qing emperor, Kangxi, confronted Galdan in battle and defeated him in the 1690s. Although Galdan died in 1697, possibly a victim of poisoning by his own people, the Qing had only temporarily ended the Jungar threat in the northwest.

In the middle of the eighteenth century, a new generation of western Mongol leaders once more challenged the Qing. This time, Qing troops were dispatched in greater numbers to the northwest, their goal being to "pacify" the region. As part of this campaign, the Qing court sought the assistance of another enemy of the western Mongols—the Kazak confederation, just to the west of Jungar lands.

At the time of the eighteenth century Qing-Oyrat wars, the Kazaks were fighting to retain control of pastures throughout Central Eurasia. In the west they contended with expanding Russian authority; to the east they fought the encroaching Mongols. Guiding the Kazaks in this difficult period was one of the last great Kazak khans, Ablai, who represents an important link in the Kazaks' future relationship with China.

Ablai was born in 1711 in what is now Kazakstan, and his original name was Abul Mansur. His family were minor nobility, tracing their descent back five generations to Jangir Khan of the Mongol Chagatai branch. According to Kazak tradition, the five generations were Jangir Khan, Wali Bala, Ablai, Wali, and Abul Mansur (Ablai). Ablai's grandfather had been ruler of the Kazak Orta Juz (Middle Horde). When Ablai was still a child, Oyrats attacked his family, killing his father and forcing the family to flee westward in 1723.[9]

As a young man, Ablai allied himself to senior Kazak leaders, the first of which was Tulibiji (Tuliebijia) of the Great Horde, for whom he pastured camels and then horses. Various sources contend that Ablai became a khan of the Great Horde, a title he retained during his rise to power in the Middle Horde. He later joined forces with one of the great leaders of the Middle Horde, Abul Mambet, to whom he was related through his grandfather and with whom he fought the Oyrat in the 1720s and 1730s. It was during this time that his name was changed to Ablai.[10] As a result of his ability, he was elected a sultan of the Middle Horde, probably by 1730. In 1733 Semeke, khan of the Middle Horde, died; Ablai and Abul Mambet then shared leadership of the Middle Horde, with the aging Abul gradually leaving more and more of the administration of the horde to Ablai.[11] While Kazak sources accord Ablai the title of khan beginning in 1735, his title during this period appears to have been sultan.

A skilled military leader, Ablai led Kazak cavalry into battle against the Oyrats. In 1740 he commanded an army of 30,000 men, among whom were many designated as *batur* (hero), a title only earned for military prowess. In a battle in 1741, Ablai was captured by the Oyrats, under their leader Galdan Cereng. After prolonged negotiations, Ablai was set free in 1743—after which there was a period of peace on the eastern Kazak steppe.

Further west, however, there was unrest. Kazaks of the Small Horde periodically fought against or allied with the Russians, in a constant struggle over access to pastures. As early as 1731, khan of the Kazak

Small Horde, had sworn allegiance to Russia; in 1734 he agreed to pay tribute. After a brief revolt against his Russian allies in 1738, he once again renewed his allegiance, a pattern to be repeated by his Kazak successors. When Abul Khayr was finally killed by a rival, Barak, in 1748, the Small Horde came under Nur Ali Khan. Nur Ali enjoyed Russian support, but he was opposed by many Kazaks, who preferred Janibek, a rival claimant. Ablai initially agreed to join Nur Ali in a new alliance, which was comprised of Ablai's own Middle Horde, Nur Ali's Small Horde, and Ablai's former enemy, the Oyrats—all of whom were to join together in opposition to Qing expansion into Central Asia. But as the powerful Manchu military won a series of battles against the Oyrat empire, Ablai agreed to receive envoys from China, abandoning his opposition and once more becoming an enemy of the Oyrat.

By the time Ablai entered into talks and, subsequently, into a trade agreement with the Qing, he was the supreme power in the Middle Horde, clans of which pastured in Semirechiye area, where Ablai was headquartered, and in the Tarbagatay Mountains.[12] His geographic position, as well as his own independence as khan, made it imperative that he balance demands of Kazak allies, some of whom were already under protection of the Russian empire, with the increasingly powerful Manchus to the east. He appears to have done this well, playing off all sides to the advantage of both his own horde and his own position within the Kazak confederation. In 1756, the Qing grand council sent Ablai an edict, the aim of which was to prevent his alliance with Amursana, an erstwhile Qing ally who revolted in 1755 to join the Oyrats.[13] Ablai remained aloof initially, but by 1757 his representatives informed the Qing that he would pay tribute and would trade with the Qing at Ulungu, a trading point in the Tarbagatay Mountains.

Anxious not only to secure Kazak horses but also to forestall any union of the Kazak with the Oyrats' Jungar empire, the Qing welcomed the trade, but stipulated that it take place only at Urumqi, a more advantageous site for them. Trade began in 1758, when three hundred horses were traded at Urumqi.[14] Possibly reluctant to make the journey into an area dominated by the Manchu military, initially only a few Kazaks appeared to begin trade, and it was late in the year before Ablai's nephew appeared there to trade, presumably acting as a representative of his powerful uncle.[15] That same year, the Qing pacification of the Oyrat began in earnest; by 1759 not only Amursana, but also the principal Oyrat leaders had been hunted down and eliminated by Man-chu military units under General Zhaohui.[16]

With the Oyrat defeated, Qing-Kazak trade expanded. The Ili River valley soon replaced Urumqi as a commercial center, trade having begun there as early as 1760. The Manchu town of Ili became the headquarters for Qing rule in the northwest regions, and garrison de-mands for locally bred horses as military mounts led to increased trade with Kazaks. At Ili, the Chinese paid two or three taels (a silver cur-rency) per horse—a bargain in comparison to the eight taels a horse cost in the closest Chinese province of Gansu. Bringing animals across the Gobi to the northwest added greatly to the cost as it increased the risk of animals dying in the desert wastes.

To encourage Kazaks to bring their animals to Ili, the Chinese would pay the best prices there. Trade also began at Tarbagatay, a trading point authorized by the Qing in 1763. Tarbagatay was a more advantageous market for Kazaks of the Middle Horde, whose pastures were close by.[17] Unauthorized trade also occurred in several places in Jungaria, despite Qing attempts to control it.

Trade goods consisted of Kazak horses, oxen, and sheep; in return, Kazaks bought medium-grade Chinese silk, satin, and cotton cloth. According to James Millward's recent study, tea played a relatively minor role in the Kazak-Manchu trade relationship. Kazaks bought or traded for tea from Mongols—who had established regularized trade with prosperous Shanxi merchants.[18]

In the 1760s, Kazaks began to use winter camps in what the Qing considered their territory, as indicated by border markers. For this privilege they paid tax to the Qing, at the rate of 1 percent of their herd. In spring, the Kazaks were obliged to move west, out of Jungaria; but poorer Kazaks, resisting attempts to make them move on, returned to the winter pastures in summer months. As did other peoples in Central Asian lands, the Kazaks raided herds to recoup losses, taking both cattle and horses—a practice that increased Qing concerns about Kazak access to the now-depopulated Jungar lands. Thus, while some Kazaks were allowed to join the Manchus' banner system in the late 1700s, the Qing generally sought to keep Kazaks beyond the Tar-bagatay Mountain ranges.

After the Jungar defeat in 1759, relations between the Qing and the Kazaks remained complicated by the presence of the Russians. While Ablai had in principle agreed to pay tribute to the Qing, and had been entered onto the Qing rolls as a tributary of the Manchus, he also pursued a guarded relationship with Russia. In 1740 he and Abul Mambet had pledged their loyalty to Russia, but they had declined to have their titles confirmed by the Russians. With Abul Mambet's retirement in 1744, Ablai became de facto head of the Middle Horde, if not also in name. With the death of Barak, a rival claimant, in 1750, his position was unassailable; indeed, no other Kazak could challenge Ablai's preeminence among the Kazaks. As such, he was courted by the Chinese and established trade relations with them in the 1750s, as described above, even while he continued to have relations with the Russians. From 1761 to 1764 he received a grain allowance from the Russian empress Catherine. Still he managed to retain his and his people's independence from both empires.

In 1770 he was elected khan of the Great Horde, and in the following year was also formally named as khan of the Middle Horde.[19] Thus, in the 1770s, Ablai was at the height of his powers. In 1775, his son and heir, Vali, petitioned Russia for grants in aid, which Empress Catherine declined to give. As the Russian throne had not yet invested Ablai as khan, Ablai's son pressed the Russians for this honor on behalf of his father, and the Russians finally agreed. Rather than travel to Russian territory, however, Ablai insisted that the Russians travel to him. He was formally recognized by the Russian throne as khan in 1778 on his own territory. It is not clear what impact this recognition had on the Qing and its relations with the Kazaks—or, indeed, whether they even knew of this development.

When Ablai died in 1781, at the age of seventy, the era of Kazak independence was ending. His successors did not enjoy his authority or his prestige, and both the Chinese and the Russians continued to draw supporters from among the Kazaks, dividing them and strengthening their own holds on Central Asian territory. The Nayman, for instance, elected their own khan, Abul Gazi, who ruled with Chinese support. A more important split among tribes of the Middle Horde occurred when Vali, Ablai's heir, sent his own son to the Chinese in 1794–1795, offering Kazak submission as a means to counter Russian influence on the steppe. Unhappy with this move, some of the clans turned toward Russia for protection. With his power thereby diminished, Vali eventually sought protection in Chinese territory, moving into Qing territory in 1806; the Russians nominated Bukei Khan as his successor. Vali's death in 1817 was followed by the death of Bukei Khan in 1818, giving the Russians an opportunity to replace Kazak governing structures with their own. Russia had already established a special tribunal in 1798 to handle disputes on the steppes; and despite the tribunal's lack of success (Kazaks would not bring any cases for its adjudication), it represented a step toward replacing traditional Kazak institutions. In 1822, the Russians made further changes in steppe administration, and in 1824 they formally abolished the title of khan, refusing to invest any further leaders with the title.[20]

Such moves did not improve Russia's relations with Ablai's heirs. His son Sarzhan actively opposed expanding Russian power on the steppes; upon Sarzhan's death in 1836, his half brother, Kenisary Kasimov, continued armed opposition. In 1838, Kenisary demanded that the khan title be restored. At the head of some 20,000 men, he disrupted Russian trade to the extent of some 8 million rubles.[21] Kenisary was in many ways a worthy successor to Ablai, developing a Kazak law code and appointing judges and taxing caravans that traversed his lands. But his costly disruption of Russian trade led to a massive Russian counterattack, as a result of which Kenisary was forced to accept an amnesty in 1844. He and his followers then joined the Kirghiz, assisting them in their efforts to break away from the Kokand khanate. He died in the fighting in 1847.

Within Chinese territory, individual Kazak khans and princes became Qing subjects for short periods in the eighteenth and nineteenth centuries, paying tribute as required by the authorities. Kazaks also continued to cross between Jungaria and the western steppes, trading with the Qing at Yili and other centers in Eastern Turkestan—the Qing's so-called Western Regions. The exact border between China and the Russian empire remained unclear, however, until both agreed to the Protocol of Tarbagatay, concluded October 7, 1864. Under the terms of this agreement, borders were established, and Kazaks living within the Qing territory of the Ili-based governor-general now became Qing subjects.[22]

Although the Qing's Western Region was far distant from the rulers in Beijing and was maintained by the Qing only at very considerable expense, nonetheless when rebellion threatened to tear the region away from Qing control, the court decided to expend whatever funds—and lives—were necessary to retain their position in the northwest. Thus in response to the rebellion of Yakub Beg of Kokand, who arrived in Kashgar in 1864 to liberate it from "infidel" Chinese hands and to provide Islamic rule to its Muslim population, the Qing launched an expedition that ended in Yakub Beg's death in 1877 and the reimposition of Qing control. The Qing court decided to make the entire region an administrative unit of the empire, declaring it to be the province of Xinjiang in 1884.

During Yakub Beg's rebellion, the Russians—ever watchful for opportunities in the region—occupied the whole of the Ili River valley, ostensibly to protect Russian nationals working there. Despite the Qing's general ineptitude in diplomatic matters during that time, they were nonetheless successful in forcing the withdrawal of Russia from the valley and in reasserting their claim over these lands.

Toward the end of the nineteenth century, both China and Russia clearly had an interest in maintaining stability along what was now a lengthy shared border. Throughout this period, however, Kazaks from the Russian side continued to enter Eastern Turkestan. For example, in 1878 not less than 9,000 Kazaks left Russian territory for China. Many of them tried to go as far as the town of Qitai. The Russian explorer N.M. Przhevalsky saw many rotting carcasses left by Kazak herds that had succumbed to thirst during the move through the Jungarian desert.[23]

There were various reasons motivating such risky undertakings. After the abolition of serfdom in Russia in 1861, Russian peasants started to move eastward, settling and farming in Central Eurasia. More than 500 villages had been established on the steppe by the end of the nineteenth century, aided by a czarist commission of 1895 that provided funds for new settlers on lands that had been used mainly by Kazak nomads. The increasing number of Russian and Ukrainian peasants on the Kazak plain became an important factor in the continual migration of Kazaks into East Turkestan.

But Russian colonization and settlement was not the only cause of Kazak migration into Chinese territory. Political unrest and Russian claims on Chinese lands also pushed the Kazaks away from the immediate border area. Kazaks started to move into the Barkol area in eastern Jungaria in 1883, when the second Tarbagatay treaty between Russia and China was signed that year. The first group of about ninety households left the uncertainty of pastures in the Altay and Tarbagatay ranges, which were on the border between China and Russia, for the relative safety of Barkol. They were followed in 1895 by another two hundred Kazak households from Altay.[24]

At the beginning of the twentieth century, the Kazaks in China were concentrated primarily in the farthest northwestern districts of the new province of Xinjiang. They were administered through a hierarchy established by the Manchu government, which included *ambans* responsible for each of the districts bordering Russia. While such officials ruled with the authority of the Qing, control in Kazak areas still remained in the hands of the traditional Kazak elite—whose titles were now confirmed by the Manchu rulers in Beijing. Rather than that of khan, the Manchus conferred the title of *wang* (prince) on important leaders. They also conferred the generic title of *taiji* (chieftain). Below the taiji were *mingbasi,* chiefs of one thousand; below those, *juzbasi,* chiefs of one hundred. These titles and their units of ten families were similar to the system of *bao jia,* which had long been used in China as a supplementary administrative system for control at the village level. The goal was to divide the nomadic groups into administrative units and to distribute political power between the different tribal segments. A taiji therefore had the dual function of lineage leader and of Qing official. The result was a relatively stable administrative system with far-reaching autonomy for the various lineage groups, but which also worked to the advantage of the Qing. Other traditional titles continued in use, including *batur,* a nonhereditary title earned only on the battlefield; *tore,* indicating nobility and descent from one of the Kazaks' great khans such as Ablai; and Muslim titles such as *hakim* (judge); *hoja* (teacher); *imam,* signifying a religious teacher; and *mullah,* a religious leader. The court-conferred titles gave great authority to those who received them. Even after the 1911 revolution brought an abrupt end to the Manchu-imposed system of titles and rewards, some families continued to use these titles until 1949.

By the end of the nineteenth century, the Qing dynasty was beset by the many challenges that would bring an end to China's imperial period. The Manchus had more than doubled the territory to which they had succeeded in 1644, and the population of imperial lands had risen from 150 million to nearly 400 million people. The dual pressures of expanded territory—which had to be both protected and administered—and massive population growth contributed to systemic collapse. Despite the great importance of the 1912 republican revolution for Chinese society, however, administration of the far northwest remained deeply rooted in past Chinese practices and attitudes.

Before turning to the Kazaks in republican China (1912–1949)—an era of revolution for the Chinese and of great upheaval for Kazaks living within China's borders—we turn to an account of Kazak culture and social organization. The forms of organization and cultural practices described below continued into the early 1950s, at which point it becomes difficult to chart changes in Kazak areas because of very limited and heavily government-mediated sources—a situation that improved only after the death of Mao in 1976. We will return to aspects of Kazak culture in contemporary society in chapter 6.

Kazak Social History, Nineteenth and Twentieth Centuries

From their beginnings as a political entity in the sixteenth century under the Kazak khanate, the Kazaks have been Muslim. Profession of faith, observance of Muslim practices in everyday life, and self-identification as Muslims—as distinct from the nonbelievers of both Russian and Chinese civilizations—have marked the Kazaks as members of greater Islamic civilization for centuries.

Despite the Kazaks' centuries-long commitment to Islam, Western accounts of Kazak culture invariably describe the Kazaks as nominal Muslims, a depiction that often accompanies discussion of the Kazaks as backward or simple folk, who are thereby incapable of the supposedly deeper religious commitment evinced by other, more devout Muslim communities. Leaving aside for the moment how one would define a devout community, it is important to note the sources for this image of Kazak religious belief. Much of it can be traced to upperclass European explorers of the mid to late nineteenth century and to a small number of trained ethnographers, both of which groups consistently described the Kazaks as nominal Muslims. Nineteenth-century observers like British Colonel Forsythe and the Earl of Dunmore and Russians such as A.N. Kuropatkin and N.M. Przhevalsky noted that the Kazaks appeared to be the least observant of all Muslims, most reportedly never having seen a mosque and few having a *madrasa,* or religious, education. Isolated from the great Islamic centers of learning and with little or no access to religious teachers or leaders who might enforce the observance of Muslim practices, their collective Kazak laxity in following the Five Pillars of Islam has been described as understandable, as was Kazak illiteracy—yet another factor noted in these accounts as distancing Kazaks from more orthodox Muslim peoples. Such depictions have continued to influence modern scholarship.[25]

Only recently have such characterizations been challenged. Devin DeWeese's recent study of conversion narratives in Central Eurasian history notes that for Inner Asian peoples Islam was "both transformative and . . . attuned to pre-Islamic traditions."[26] He asserts that conversion narratives such as that of Baba Tukles—who, according to traditional narratives, converted Özbek Khan to Islam in the early fourteenth century—illustrate the ways in which the Islamic faith was articulated among the ordinary Turkic-speaking peoples of the steppe. He draws overdue attention to the many indicators of Islamic influence in everyday life among the Kazak and other steppe nomads, including the adoption of Muslim personal and communal names, Muslim self-designation, adoption of Muslim rituals such as ablution and daily prayer, circumcision, Muslim methods of slaughter, and so on.

DeWeese also reminds us of the importance of the spoken word in preliterate society. In the steppe world, where binding agreements relied on oral rather than written records, the spoken word carried great power—power that could be at once magical and sacred, binding and eternal. Words were power, and in steppe societies one did not speak lightly of important matters. As Dale Eickelman and James Piscatori have pointed out, there has been an almost unquestioned assumption that a written record is more powerful than an oral tradition. Print-centered European cultures have, as a result, been dismissive of those societies in which oral forms have been the primary means of recording and interpreting the past as well as the primary means through which to understand and articulate religious belief. Eickelman and Piscatori also note that, in any case, interpretation and understanding of the Koran and other sacred texts depend on "the political, social and economic circumstances of those interpreting them."[27] Thus the lack of print technology or great material wealth does not render an oral culture less able to understand or interpret religious ideas, nor should its members be viewed as less religious because of the absence of religious texts.

The importance of words and oral tradition are clearly reflected in the Kazak emphasis on knowledge of one's genealogy for five preceding generations. This knowledge was an intrinsic part of membership in Kazak society, providing a particular, individual identity and positioning a person within clan and Juz. A person's name would thus not only be a signifier of membership in the group, but would also link him or her to the group's collective past. In some parts of China, the practice of reciting the names of five generations of ancestors is still a method of identification between Kazaks meeting for the first time. Having the names of Muslim saints as well as descendants of Chinggis Khan among one's earliest ancestors has also remained a source of great honor and family prestige.

Ultimately, as DeWeese notes, from a Muslim viewpoint, there can be no "nominal" adoption of Islam: One either accepts the tenets of the religion or one doesn't. The depths of a person's religious devotion is not a matter for others to assess, but lies in the mind of the individual believer. As noted in the discussion of Kazak cultural history that follows, Islam has been so integral a part of Kazak society that from the earliest history of the Kazak khanate to the present, being Kazak has also meant being Muslim.

Social Organization

Historically, the Kazaks consisted of pastoral tribes of mixed Turkic and Mongolian origin that united in confederations in the fifteenth and sixteenth centuries, as described above. From these origins, the Kazaks developed into a consolidated ethnic unit. Kazaks at the end of the twentieth century still consider themselves to be divided into three hordes, commonly referred to as the Great, or Large, Horde (in Kazak, Ulu Juz); the Middle, or Central, Horde (Orta Juz); and the Lesser, or Small, Horde (Kishi Juz).

Like other nomadic groups of Central Eurasia, the Kazaks' social organization is based on descent groups. All three of the hordes are subdivided into kinship units, called *uru,* which can also be classified as maximal lineages. In Xinjiang, a majority of the Kazaks are of the Middle Horde, which is further divided into six uru: Kerey, Nayman, Waq, Kongrat, Qipchaq, and Arghin. Only the first three were represented in Xinjiang during the first half of the century. Although detailed information on the organization of the Middle Horde is scant, the location of and relations between the uru in Xinjiang can be traced, as can the lineages most important among Xinjiang Kazaks.

In the nineteenth century, the Kerey pastured their animals in the valley of the Kara Irtish River and in the southern Altay Mountains. By the mid-twentieth century, the Kerey were the single largest lineage in Xinjiang, with pastures in the Altay and along the Irtish Valley and also in the Tian Shan. Smaller numbers were distributed in other parts of Jungaria, near Bogda Ulu and Lake Barkol. The Nayman had their pastures on the west bank of the Irtish River as well as in the valley of the Kara Irtish, the Tarbagatay basin, and the lands surrounding Murka Kol. By the middle of the twentieth century, they reportedly lived in the Emil River valley and in mountainous areas within the Tarbagatay district. The less numerous Waq Kazaks were dispersed in small contingents among the Kerey and Nayman. By the 1990s, groups from all three uru were to be found distributed throughout Xinjiang, as well as in the former republics of the Soviet Union and in the Mongolian People's Republic.

Each uru is divided into many subgroups, which are also usually called uru, although the term *el* is also used to describe them.[28] The lineages are named after a fictive, or mythic, ancestor, and lineage members respect their relationship through practices such as exogamy.

The Kerey consisted of twelve lineages, namely Jantekey, Jadiq, Iteli, Merkit, Molqi, Jastabaw, Kongsadaq, Shiymoyin, Shibarajghur, Qaraqas, Sarbas, and Sherwsu. Although all the lineages are regarded as equal, the Jantekey is subdivided into additional lineages, which are regarded as equivalent to the original twelve, or the Oneki Kerey lineages.

The Nayman of Xinjiang are divided into nine lineages, which are the Tortuwil, Sadir, Matay, Qaragerey, Ergenekti, Baghanali, Kokjarli, Sarjomart, and Terstangbali. These are said to constitute the "nine dawn sons of the Nayman," according to Kazaks.[29] In addition, Xinjiang Nayman informants report the Musqali, Bura, Beyjighit, and Aqnayman as lineages represented in Xinjiang during the twentieth century. As in the past, the lineages remain a source of an individual Kazak's sense of belonging and identity.

Political and Administrative Structure

The extent to which the Kazaks have had a single, unified administrative system or political leadership remains uncertain. The lineages, described briefly above, provided a sense of identity and continuity with the past, but neither the lineages nor the larger uru functioned as administrative units during the Chinese republic.

In the twentieth century, vestiges of the Qing system of administration remained in the Kazak areas. The Qing title of wang, for example, remained a nominal part of Kazak society. One prominent Kerey Kazak leader, Alin Wang, resided in Urumqi under the Chinese republic. In the Chinese view, he was a principal leader of the Kazak tribes; in fact, his power and influence were negligible.

After the 1912 revolution, northern Xinjiang was divided into five districts (aymaq), four of which had Kazaks as the district head (aymaq bastiq) by the 1940s. Each district was subdivided into a county, each of which was—theoretically—administered by a county chief (taiji). During the 1940s, there were some thirty taiji in Xinjiang. More important in the day-to-day affairs of most Kazaks were local chiefs or leaders; these included the mingbasi (or okurday) who was responsible for 300 to 600 yurts, or households; the juzbasi, who led 100 to 100 yurts; and the onbasi, leading 10 to 30 yurts.[30] The system was inconsistent, however, with some districts having men at each of these levels and others having only one or two ranks filled. For example, during the days of the warlord Sheng, Urumqi district had men holding the ranks of taiji, okurday, and juzbasi, while the Altay districts kept much of the old Manchu system. Until 1949, the leaders of each Kazak district were appointed by the authorities in Urumqi, while the lower-level leaders were usually men who had inherited their positions.[31]

Marriage and Household

The Xinjiang Kazak household could be either a conjugal or an extended-family unit. As mentioned above, Kazak lineages are exogamous; repeated marriages between two lineages created closer ties between them, and Kazaks in such relationships refer to each other as sarsuyek quda [yellowbone relative]. Marriages between Kazaks and other Muslim groups were acceptable, although there are no figures available on the frequency of such marriages.

There were several ways of choosing spouses among the Kazaks. Prior to 1949, parents arranged the marriages of their children, but the parties could object. Young people being pressured into marriage were also known to take matters into their own hands and elope.[32] Marriages generally took place just after puberty for girls and in the midteens for boys.

Traditionally, the groom paid a bride-price (qalim), provided by his family and, in some instances, by his kin. The bride brought a dowry to the marriage, usually including a yurt, household goods, and livestock. Customary law decreed that such goods could not be disposed of without the wife's consent and were therefore not a part of the husband's patrimony.[33]

If a family was poor and unable to afford the bride-price, a man could be in his thirties before being able to arrange for a wife. One custom that allowed families to avoid the system of bride-price and dowry was the exchange of brides (*qarsi qudaliq*), in which two families would exchange daughters as brides for their respective sons.

Marriage celebrations were joyous occasions, celebrated with enthusiasm and marked by various festivities. No other transition rite could compete with the marriage in its richness and complexity. It included a ritualized performance of matchmaking, the offering of the bride-price (*qalim mal*), the presentation of the dowry (*jasaw*), repeated reciprocal exchanges of gifts, the singing of laments, and the ceremonial removal of the bridal veil (*betasar*).[34] In addition, weddings were the occasion of horseback racing, feasts (*toy*), and drinking fermented mare's milk, kumiss. Kazaks followed patrilocal residence patterns and after marriage the young couple settled in the summer camp (*awil*) of the husband.

During the summer months, Kazak camps were set up in a semicircle with the yurt of the most important leader placed in the center. If such a man had more than one wife, as was allowed under Muslim practice, each woman would have her own yurt (*uy*) placed nearby. Next were the married sons' yurts (*otaw*) each with a prefix to indicate seniority; ülkü otaw, the eldest son's yurt; *ortanci otaw*, the middle son's yurt; *kiši otaw,* the youngest son's yurt—and so on. Yurts of relatives in the same lineage were placed to right of the leader's yurt (ülkün uy) while collateral relatives were placed on the left. If a religious leader, such as an imam, were traveling with the awil, his yurt would be near that of the leader. Respected guests and visiting traders were also honored in this way.[35]

While the vast majority of Kazak households included only the husband and wife, some influential Kazak leaders had several wives. According to Frank Bessac, among Xinjiang Kazaks in 1950, it was thought only proper for a man of high status to have more than one wife. The leader Osman Batur was reportedly persuaded to take a younger wife, but his strong attachment to his senior (first) wife led to his neglecting the second, eventually causing her to leave him.[36]

Despite this example, however, divorce was much easier for the man, as in many traditional, patriarchal societies. A woman could be divorced for adultery, lack of respect, disobedience, and infertility. However, divorce, like the practice of taking more than one wife, appears to have been rare in Xinjiang Kazak society.

As new members of the household, Kazak brides were expected to observe avoidance behavior, especially with regard to the older male relatives of the husband. A woman would avoid using personal names, instead using a euphemism or title. Further, if her mother-in-law or father-in-law entered the room and did not invite her to remain, she would leave.

Despite such a code of etiquette, women nonetheless held strong positions within the immediate family. Married women joined in discussions and in final decisions affecting the household. During the 1940s, at least one Kazak woman rose to a position of political power: Alin Wang's wife, Hadewan (Kadvan Hanim), became the district officer for Urumqi under the Guomindang (GMD). After 1949, she and her family changed their allegiance to the Chinese Communist Party (CCP) and remained important figures under the new government.

Migratory Cycle of Xinjiang Kazaks

The pattern of migration in evidence among the Kazaks in Xinjiang could best be described as vertical, in contrast to the horizontal pattern of Kazaks further to the west. In Xinjiang, winter pastures were in the valleys or on the Jungarian steppe; in spring, herds and flocks were moved up into the mountains. This pattern is closer to that seen among the Kirghiz, rather than that common to Kazaks on the Kazak steppe beyond Xinjiang. During these migrations, a Kazak household would move in an *awil*, or a group of households related by kinship ties. Each was led by an *awil bastiq*, or awil leader, who was responsible for such matters as deciding when and where to move and, as needed, for communicating important matters to the next highest level and to other awils.

Awils varied in size. Although most tended to be small, some could have as many as twenty households together with 4,000–5,000 sheep, 300–800 horses, 80–100 cattle, and 60–200 camels.

Wealthy Kazak leaders could afford to hire herdsmen to care for their animals. In the Ili Valley, Kazaks sometimes hired Mongols to do this work. Some of the wealthiest leaders chose to settle in towns or villages, retaining almost feudal ties with poorer herdsmen, who raised animals for them in return for a share in the herd.

Kazak winter pastures (*qistaw*) were often on or near the banks of rivers. Nearby forests provided logs for the construction of houses used by some Kazaks during the winter months. Various groups had the right to winter pastures in certain prime areas, leaving other groups the marginal areas near marshes or elsewhere. Early spring was the most critical time for the herds, for fodder could be scarce in the harsh winter climate of northern Xinjiang. A sudden late-winter or early-spring snowstorm could decimate a herd. Owners of large herds proportionally suffered the greatest losses, since those with smaller herds could manage to feed more of their animals with stored fodder. Such catastrophes, known as *jut,* led to increases in the price of meat, sometimes doubling the cost of lamb.

Kazaks left their winter pastures when the first grass began to grow. In the Tian Shan ranges, migrations could begin at the end of March or in early April; further north, in the Altay Mountains, migration began later. The first destination was the spring pastures (*köktew*), commonly a fixed place used by the same group over a period of years and located on the lower slopes of mountain ranges. The migration was a dramatic event, as observed by Owen Lattimore, an American who traveled in the Kazak areas of Xinjiang in the late 1920s:

> To force a way through the snow, they drove their pony herds before them, to trample out a rough road. Then came the oxen and cows, every one of them laden, some with felts and household furniture. Some served as saddle beasts, and often a baby would be strapped in its rough cradle on top of the load. The pony herd was in the charge of the youngest and most active men, and the cattle were guided mostly by women. After them came more men in charge of the camels, which floundered with difficulty through the frozen, slippery snow, often falling into drifts and having to be dug and hauled out. The camels, being the strongest and tallest of the animals, were laden with the poles and framework of the yurts, the round felt tents. At this time of year, the baby camels, only a few months old, are unable to stand the hardship of long difficult marches; each was tied on top of the load carried by its mother. Last of all came the great flocks of sheep, struggling and floundering through the snow. They were herded along by young boys and

girls, riding young oxen and ponies; and the saddle of every child was draped, fore and aft, with exhausted lambs picked out of the snow.[37]

At the köktew, the Kazaks branded their animals. Every household or migratory group had its own brand (*tangba*) to mark ownership. Individual animals of each member had their own mark (*en*). The larger animals were branded on their flanks with branding irons; camels were branded on their chests. The sheep and goats were marked by cuts on their ears, made with large scissors. In Kazak, these cuts are named according to the place on the ear where they are made (e.g., *kiyik en, solaw en, kez en*, etc.).

In May or early June, the next move is made, this time to higher altitudes where the Kazaks have their summer pastures (*jaylaw*). Some groups moved once more during July. Many of the pastures were marked in some way, by a stone pillar or a pile of stones. Conflict over the right to use a particular pasture was relatively common and a major source of disputes between various awils. The herds spent the summers in the mountains, growing fat on the mountain grass. During summer, animals were milked, and a range of diary products were produced by the women. Clothing and tools were also traditionally made during this season.

In the traditional division of labor, men did most of the herding, guarding the herds and moving them from pasture to pasture. They also gelded, branded, and butchered livestock, as well as milked the mares. Boys were trained in all these activities from the time they were able to walk. Occasionally, herdsmen rode into nearby towns to buy provisions of various kinds, particularly supplies of salt for the sheep, but also for tea, sugar, and household items they could not manufacture themselves, such as iron cooking pots. Much of the work around the camp and in the yurt was the domain of women. Among myriad other chores, they cooked; gathered firewood and dung for fuel; milked cows, sheep, and camels; took care of the children; made clothing and shoes; and helped produce felt.

During the summertime, the Kazak diet consisted of meat and milk products. The latter included kumiss (*qimiz*) and sour milk (*ayran*). In addition, women made products such as *qatiq*, a kind of cottage cheese; *qurt*, dried cheese curds; and *irimshiq* and *aq irimshiq*, hard, dry cheeses. Salted tea was prepared repeatedly throughout the day, and flat bread was a part of most meals. Meat was eaten more regularly in the summer months than at other times, although the poorer Kazaks relied on cereals, saving their animals in order to build their herds. Vegetables were rare, except for root crops such as onion or garlic. The main meal was eaten in the evening.

Hunting provided both additional sources of food as well as recreation for the men. The preferred game included deer, mountain sheep, fox, wolves, and game birds. Some Kazaks specialized as hunters, and the furs and pelts they gathered brought high prices in the local markets. Hunters from the Altay told one of the authors about even more exotic game. During a hunting expedition in the 1930s, two men of the Shaqabay lineage captured a *qiiq adam,* or wild man, which they brought back to their camp. The furious hairy creature clawed people, so they tied it to a pole near their yurt. Since it appeared to have breasts, they decided it must be female. All night the creature cried wildly, and by morning they felt so sorry for it that they released her.

At the end of the summer, awils started to move back to winter pastures. Reversing the spring movement, they moved down to lower autumn pastures (*kuzin*), where the sheep were sheared. Once back in the winter pasture, some animals were sold, while others were slaughtered for the Kazaks' own consumption.

Despite the fact that some Kazaks settled in Jungaria and a few made their living as smiths, saddle makers, carpenters, and even fishermen, the majority of Kazaks remained pastoral nomads. Seeing their herds increase in number, acquiring many horses, and hunting with friends constituted the optimal conditions for a satisfying life to Kazak men. Cultural values associated with this independent lifestyle included admiration for bravery, for martial skills, and for freedom from the restrictions that, in the Kazak view, marked the lives of those living in towns and settlements. Every Kazak male was a potential warrior, ready to defend the honor of his family and the well-being of his animals with his life. Those who were successful in these endeavors earned remembrance in folk songs and stories, continuing the oral tradition of honoring heroes. The title of batur was conferred on those who could claim leadership in battle and the loyalty of men willing to follow them whatever the odds. Bravery could also be demonstrated through raids to acquire animals to build both the herds and the stature of those participating. Horses were especially prized; the term *barimta* referred to horse theft, which was deemed warranted in certain circumstances. For example, if a man did not obtain a girl promised as his wife from another lineage group, a raid for horses from that group was seen as justified.

Kazak Livestock

The basis of the Kazak family's economy was the sheep, the primary source of food and family income. Kazaks in Xinjiang relied on the fat-tailed sheep for milk, mutton, wool, and leather. A few goats were often kept with the sheep, as herd leaders and for searching out grass, something they were better at than the sheep. This practice was common among sheepherding peoples all over Central Asia, and continues in Xinjiang today, particularly among Kazaks at Bogda Ulu. In addition to leading the herds, goats were also milked.

Although the sheep are vital to the family, the horse remained the animal with the highest status among the Kazaks. Horses were kept for riding, for transport, for meat and milk, and for sale. In the summer, young horses and stallions grazed the meadows, while the mares were kept near the yurts. About twenty mares were kept for each stallion. Mares could be milked up to five times a day, a task usually performed by men, although occasionally women performed this task. Horse flesh was a highly prized meat, and horse-meat sausage was considered a great delicacy. Another dish featuring horse-meat was a kind of stew, *qouwirdaq*. Horses from Barkol, the Ili Valley, and Karashar (Yanqi) were highly prized and widely sought in markets all over the region.

Some Kazaks also kept horned cattle, for milk and hides as well as to employ as beasts of burden. In the Ili Valley, where cattle could winter with relative safety, large numbers were kept throughout the summer months and then sold in the autumn.

Camels also played a role in the Kazak diet; but they, too, were milked and used for transport or to carry household goods, particularly the various components of the yurt. While the Chinese and Mongols pierce the camel for the bit below and well back from the opening of the nostril, the Kazaks did it above the level of the nostrils, where the cartilage is said to be much weaker. Xinjiang Kazaks tended to keep few camels, however. As they are steppe animals, it was difficult to keep them at the higher altitudes in the mountains during the summers. Kazaks who kept camels sometimes specialized in breeding them, selling the animals to the Chinese and the Uyghurs as beasts of burden.

Another common domestic animal was the dog. There were two

breeds, one to guard the stock from predators and a breed of grey-hound, the *taz it*, used for hunting. Kazaks also used eagles for hunting: A good hunting eagle could cost the same as two of the best horses. Skill with these majestic birds was admired, and the very best birds were commonly not sold but bestowed on chieftains and other high-ranking persons as a sign of honor.

By the early twentieth century, the Kazaks of Xinjiang remained at the margins of the Chinese empire. Although technically a part of the new Chinese republic, which began on January 1, 1912, they continued to follow traditional patterns of life, following their herds and obeying their own traditional leaders with little regard to the greater political changes that would soon draw them into the tumultuous twentieth century.

— 3 —

China's Kazaks,
1912-1949

The Chinese revolution of 1911 ended the Qing dynasty but did not end Chinese rule in Xinjiang. Instead, it ushered in a period of Chinese warlord rule that ended in rebellion and the secession of three of the province's ten districts, which formed their own independent state in 1944. Thus the first half of the twentieth century saw the region move from colonial outpost, through successive Chinese warlord regimes, to partial independence, being incorporated into the PRC in 1949.

Before turning to the role of warlords and revolutionaries in Kazak affairs during this period, we will first examine the basic policies that evolved in the republican era for minority areas like Xinjiang. Lack of power to implement policy in the border regions did not prevent the central government from formulating policies. These formulations indicate not only the general direction that GMD policy would eventually take, but also the beliefs and attitudes of many government officials toward minority populations. In the 1940s, when GMD control was finally introduced to Xinjiang, the strongly paternalistic and authoritarian attitudes of the men sent to govern the region continued to complicate Han-Muslim relations. A discussion of GMD policy also reveals strong continuity between policies of the GMD and the CCP— for despite their ideological differences, the parties agreed on such key elements as the necessity for Chinese-led economic development in minority areas and the need to introduce large numbers of Han Chinese settlers into border regions of strategic importance.

From the beginning, the Chinese republic recognized China's multi-ethnic composition. The earliest clear indication of this can be seen in Dr. Sun Yatsen's references to China's "five nationalities." He asserted that five great peoples comprised the greater Chinese nation: Manchus, Mongols, Muslims, Tibetans, and, of course, the majority Han Chinese. The term *nationality* suggests an acceptance of separate national identities; but as Sun's writings indicate, the five peoples were all considered to be fundamentally Chinese. Differences in physical characteristics, language, religion, and culture were seen as resulting from the relative historical isolation of these groups from the majority of the Chinese over many centuries. Given these views, it reasonably followed that Sun envisaged a time when all such differences and cultural distinctions would die out, when a new, single nation would arise by a kind of reassimilation, absorbing the peoples who had become separated from the ethnic core of Han Chinese. The new nation would then "satisfy the demands and requirements of all races and unite them in a single cultural and political whole."[1]

Four "minority" groups were thus included among the five elemental Chinese nationalities. This was of great political import as a defense of the new state's claim to the territory of the former Qing dynasty. The Manchu rulers of the Qing had had a special relationship with both the Mongols and Tibetans dating from preconquest times (pre-1644). This relationship had, furthermore, been strengthened many times over by intermarriage between elite Mongol families and the Manchu's ruling Aisin Gioro clan and by the imperial favor shown to Tibetan Buddhism, particularly from the eighteenth century on. More recent was China's mid-eighteenth-century conquest of the far northwest, ending in the Qing creation of the new province of Xinjiang in 1884. All these areas, however, remained outside the core area of Chinese civilization, and very few Chinese lived beyond the Great Wall to the north of Beijing or west of the Gobi or on the Tibetan plateau. Thus the early republic's recognition of the indigenous peoples of these lands was at once a recognition of their special relationship to the last dynasty and a declaration of the need to preserve the republic's inherited territorial base. As successor to the Manchu empire, the republic took responsibility for all the territories of the Qing and for all the peoples who inhabited them. That such expansiveness was motivated less by concern for minority sensibilities than by a desire to confirm China's rights can be seen in the republic's privileging of these "nationalities" over far more numerous non-Han populations, such as the Chuang, Yi, or Miao peoples—all of whom were significantly greater in number than the Tibetans or Mongols, but whose lands were not seen as susceptible to dismemberment by interfering outside powers.

The early republic had limited government machinery to deal with its predominantly non-Han areas. Initially, the primary institution for all minority affairs was the Ministry of Mongolian and Tibetan Affairs, a holdover from the Qing that was directly responsible to the president.[2] In 1928, the ministry was reorganized and renamed the Mongolian and Tibetan Affairs Commission, with the status of a ministry under the executive Yuan.[3]

The most important—indeed, perhaps the only—function of the commission was planning. Various schemes for the economic development of the border areas were drawn up, based on reports of officials sent to explore the potential resources of these areas.[4] These reports stressed the need for economic development along with improved transportation and communication, the poor state of which constituted a barrier to the closer integration of border regions with China proper. The natural resources of areas like Xinjiang were of special interest. In the 1930s extensive planning was begun for the future exploitation of this wealth, plans that, it was hoped, would be implemented once government control could be established.

During the Nanjing decade (1928–1937), Chiang Kaishek's government hoped to make use of the riches of these areas, but the necessary control proved to be elusive. In Xinjiang, the central government was only able to forge a tenuous connection to the region's new warlord, General Sheng Shicai.

Although still powerless to implement policy during Sheng's rule, which lasted from 1933 to 1944, the Nationalist government expressed concern for more than just the region's potential wealth by establishing provincial-level departments of the Mongolian and Tibetan Education Department, which, despite the name, was charged with overseeing the development of education among all of China's minorities. A major feature of these education programs was the promotion of an understanding of the Chinese nation and the responsibilities of citizenship.[5]

Teaching the Chinese language to all minorities was also a fundamental part of policy on paper until 1945, when this requirement was no longer stressed; after all, as the government by then freely admitted, little headway had been made in teaching Chinese to any of the non-Han peoples in China.[6] High rates of illiteracy remained the rule in most minority regions.

Another important area of Nationalist policy was the planned resettlement of Han Chinese in minority areas. Although the central government could do little more than plan for the future, on a few occasions the government attempted to settle Chinese peasants in Xinjiang. Only small groups were involved prior to 1949, and the results of these relocations were often disastrous for the peasants involved. For example, in 1943, over 4,000 refugees from Henan arrived in Xinjiang. They were promised land, but as a result of local mismanagement, most became tenants or hired hands.[7]

During the republican era, the major concern of the government with regard to all border and minority areas was to secure these lands as integral parts of the state. Although policy was bolstered by the belief that the non-Chinese indigenous people of these regions were "basically Chinese," in reality the government was well aware of the vulnerability of these areas to foreign intervention precisely because the populations were not Han. The need to maintain Chinese territorial integrity was combined with the rhetoric of the five nations of China to preclude granting self-determination to any non-Han peoples. Since official policy maintained that they were all basically Chinese, minorities and their lands were thus a part of the "motherland." There was, therefore, no basis for any demands for self-determination. All lands inhabited by minority populations—which amounted to over 60 percent of China's total territory—were viewed by Chiang and his supporters as an indivisible part of the Chinese state, to be governed in accord with central government's policy and to be used for the betterment of the greater Chinese nation. It followed that these people were also subject to the same laws as all other Chinese. Only Mongolia and Tibet were accorded the special recognition of having a commission bearing their names. Even in this instance, however, recognition of special status did not imply any future separate from the rest of China.

As noted above, between 1912 and 1949 China's weak central government rarely exercised real authority in minority areas. However, official GMD statements on minority issues and the actions of GMD officials and military in minority areas after World War II suggest that an effective policy would have relied strongly on the military and, ultimately, on the immigration of Han Chinese into these regions once government authority was established.

In warlord-ruled Xinjiang, a mix of imperial traditions and modern military methods were used to "manage" local populations. Despite the fact that the central government had virtually no authority in these regions for most of the republican period, there was nonetheless considerable continuity in the style of Chinese governance in border regions like Xinjiang. Patronizing local elites, manipulating minority relations (e.g., playing one minority off against another in a modern form of *yi yi zhi yi* [using barbarians to fight barbarians]), overtaxing, requisitioning goods, and harassing local populations remained the staples of Chinese rule. Whether by self-styled warlord or official appointed by Nanjing, local government was administered for the benefit of local rulers and the Chinese community, leading to intense animosity between rulers and ruled. This is well illustrated in the following discussion of warlord rule in Xinjiang, from Yang Cengxin through Sheng Shicai.

**Xinjiang and the Kazaks under Warlord Rule,
1912–1944**

Officially, Qing rule in Xinjiang ended with the founding of the republic on January 1, 1912. Nonetheless, the Qing-appointed governor, Yuan Dahua, suppressed the efforts of Chinese revolutionaries in the provincial capital in an effort to forestall the inevitable. With Han Chinese in other cities of the region threatening further disruptions, Yuan chose to leave Xinjiang in the spring, allowing his subordinate, Yang Cengxin, to take control of the government apparatus. China's new president, Yuan Shikai, who acceded to the presidency following President Sun's brief tenure in 1912, confirmed Yang in his position as the first republican-era governor of Xinjiang.

Originally from Yunnan, in 1899 Governor Yang had earned a *jinshi* degree, the highest level attainable through the imperial exams under the old dynasty. He served the Qing in various capacities in northwestern China, finally being assigned to Xinjiang in 1908. He rose to the post of commissioner for judicial affairs in Urumqi (then known as Dihua), so that he was well positioned to take over when his predecessor resigned. Xinjiang entered the republican era under the leadership of this Qing bureaucrat, whose autocratic style clearly reflected his years as a dynastic official.

As governor, Yang's first challenge was to deal with continued rebellion among Han Chinese in the region. His response was to negotiate a settlement, first, with a Chinese rival who was based in the Ili

Valley area and, second, with the rebellious Chinese followers of the Gelaohui (Elder Brother Society), a so-called secret society that claimed Han Chinese followers in many of the southern Tarim Basin cities. Backing up Yang's position in the negotiations was a force of some 2,000 Hui (or Tungan) soldiers, which became the basis for a provincial military of some 10,000 men. In addition to handling his Chinese rivals, Yang also forged his own policy toward the Muslim population and devised his own financing system, since the central government was unable to provide a subsidy. Yang and his Qing-trained officials maintained their positions through cooperation with local begs, men of wealth and position whose families had been allied to the Qing, serving as tax collectors and mediating between Han officials and the local people. Considering the difficulties Governor Yang faced during his tenure as Governor, he was remarkably success-ful in holding onto power.[8]

A recurring problem for Yang was dealing with the increasing Kazak population in his province. At the turn of the century, Kazaks had continued to move into Xinjiang from the neighboring Kazak steppe, joining those already on pastures in Jungaria, formerly the stronghold of the Oyrat Mongols [Jungars]. Under the Qing, the small groups of Kazaks in Xinjiang had been considered tenants of the Mongols and were required to pay grazing fees for using pastures that the Qing had assigned to Mongols. Kazaks were also considered sub-ject to the authority of the local amban, while the Mongols continued to be the titular subjects of their own princes (*wang*), who in turn were directly under the authority of the emperor.

Despite the fact that the Mongols enjoyed a special position in the region, the number of Kazaks continued to grow as a result of events in Russian Central Asia, where mass settlement of Russian peasants took place between 1906 and 1912, during Stolypin's attempts at agrarian reform. Nearly 19 million hectares of land on the Kazak steppe were set aside for the new settlers—land that had been used as pasturage for the nomads. The growing numbers of Russians drove thousands of Kazaks out of Russia and into China. A mass migration took place in 1912–1914, with most of the newcomers going to the Ili Valley, on the Sino-Russian border, and to the Altay Mountains, on the border with Mongolia. This influx clearly concerned the new governor, and he acted quickly. In 1914, he signed an agreement with the Russian con-sul in Urumqi, stipulating that Kazaks who had immigrated before July

1911 and who had remained in Xinjiang were to be granted Chinese citizenship. Kazaks arriving after that date were to be sent back to Russia. The central government in Beijing, evidently fearful that the Russians would use the repatriated Kazaks to bolster claims on the Ili area, decided that the number of repatriates should not exceed 6,000.[9]

Governor Yang also had to deal with other nomads who were a potential threat to the peace and security of his province. In response to the Chinese revolution, the Khalkha Mongols, on Xinjiang's eastern border, declared themselves independent and began their struggle for international recognition of what had been Outer Mongolia under the Qing. Like other Asian peoples, the Khalkhas wanted their own independent, sovereign state. Governor Yang responded to this by shifting his favor away from the Mongols and toward the Kazaks, in part to prevent the Mongols of Xinjiang's Jungarian region from following the example of the Khalkhas and declaring themselves independent. One result of this policy was to further the traditional animosities and competition for pasturage that had already marked Mongol-Kazak relations.

Formerly the tenants of the Mongols in the Altay, Kazaks were encouraged to retaliate against any Mongol provocation. Yang also allowed the distribution of weapons to the Kazaks, while withholding them from Mongols. Further, when Yang's control of the province became strong enough, he forced Mongols in the Altay Mountains to move west, distancing them from the Khalkhas. Kazaks took advantage of this and reportedly plundered the Altay area almost unchecked.[10] Finally, Yang allowed Kazaks previously forced out of the northern Altay to return. The original move, according to explorer Aurel Stein, had involved as many as 1,500 yurts, or Kazak households, seeking to escape the turmoil that marked the beginning of the struggle for Mongolian independence. When these exiles arrived in Qitai, however, they found that Chinese peasants were opening new agricultural lands on former pastures there; thus, many Kazaks were anxious to return to the Altay area, which Yang finally allowed them to do.[11]

Yang continued to watch developments across his borders with concern. Russian policy in Central Asia precipitated another wave of Kazak immigration in 1916. In that year, the czarist government decided to enlarge labor units by drafting Kazaks and other Muslims who had been previously exempt from such service. This led to a massive

revolt, involving over 50,000 men across the steppes and in the Fergh-
ana Valley. As a punishment, the Russian governor-general of
Turkestan, Kuropatkin, decided to drive nomads who took part in the
revolt away from their lands and to open those lands to Russian settlers. Settlement began while the revolt was still in progress. As a
result, in the year prior to the Russian Revolution, about 300,000 persons, mainly Kazaks, fled to Xinjiang. Governor Yang was anxious for
these people to return to Russian territory, not only because of the
stress they would place on local resources, but also because of their
potential threat to the security of his province. Through negotiations
with the new Soviet representatives in Urumqi, Yang managed to obtain an amnesty for the refugees if they agreed to return home. By
1918, many of them had reportedly returned to the USSR.[12]

Despite Yang's success in negotiating with the new USSR, a new
wave of migrants was precipitated by Soviet collectivization in Central
Asia. As a result of Soviet policy, many Kazaks saw their herds starve
on pastures that could no longer sustain them. Others, facing the threat
of expropriation of their animals, slaughtered their herds. During the
1920s, Kazaks moved into neighboring areas like Afghanistan and
Xinjiang. Kazaks who had crossed into China in the late nineteenth
century and had then returned to the steppe, once more arrived in
Xinjiang at the end of the 1920s; these included many Nayman Kazaks
who settled in the Ili Valley.

While Kazak movement across the international Sino-Soviet border
remained a matter of concern throughout Yang's tenure as governor,
he continued to develop strong trade relations with the USSR. Much of
this trade involved animals and animal products, in exchange for Soviet manufactured goods. Table 3.1 shows the growth of this trade,
which increased in value from 370,400 roubles in 1922 to 20,526,000
in 1927.

The most important export from Xinjiang was wool, which rose
from 2,548 tons in 1923–1924 to 5,261 tons in 1926–1927. But the
numbers of live animals being sent to the USSR also grew, to replace
losses in Kazakstan. The number of cattle sold rose from 6,292 in
1923–1924 to 13,073 in 1926–1927. In addition, trade in meat and
animal products during the same period rose from 2,053 tons to 4,269
tons. But by far the greatest growth was in the number of sheep, the
major product of the Kazak people. Trade in sheep amounted to 50,694
head in 1923–1924, and the number rose to 84,478 in 1926–1927. In

Table 3.1

Xinjiang-Soviet Trade, 1922–1926

Year	Xinjiang Exports	Xinjiang Imports	Total Value
1922	17.7	19.7	37.4
1923	219.8	41.3	261.1
1924	435.7	268.3	704.0
1925	797.1	606.9	1,404.0
1926	1,029.4	1,023.2	2,052.6

Source: Li Sheng, ed. Xinjiang dui Su (E) maoyi shi 1600–1990 [A history of Xinjiang's trade with the Soviet Union (Russia), 1600–1990] (1994), 324.
Note: Figures are given in units of 10,000 roubles.

return, the USSR sold cotton cloth, sugar, articles for everyday use, matches, and food products. Demand for all of these grew significantly. The tonnage of cotton cloth, for instance, dramatically increased from 66 tons to 1,581 tons, and sugar from 105 tons to 1,649 tons between 1923 and 1927.[13]

Altogether, trade with the USSR outweighed trade with all other parties, including China proper. In 1927, the region's total trade with India was valued (in roubles) at 4,002,000; with Afghanistan, 1,379,000; and with China, 2,676,000. In the same year, trade with the Soviet Union reached a value of 24,175,000 roubles.[14] Yang's tenure in Xinjiang was undoubtedly buttressed by the increasing availability of imported goods as well as by the strong demand for Xinjiang's products.

Yang's assassination in 1928 was a Chinese matter, unrelated to his policy toward Kazaks. His successor, Jin Shuren, had been a member of Yang's government, and, like Yang, he was a Qing-trained official. Jin inherited a corrupt government, and he made no moves to improve the situation. He exploited land revenues—the main source of tax income for the government—to the hilt: Almost double the legal amount of tax was reportedly collected by Chinese officials in collusion with the local begs. Requisitioning of supplies—a practice long associated with official corruption and abuse of power—continued unchecked. The government continued its monopoly over gold and jade. In other areas of trade, Chinese officials reportedly dominated the market as well. According to one estimate, only 12 percent of local-trade capital belonged to local merchants, 37 percent to foreign firms, and a full 51 percent to Chinese officials and their relatives.[15]

Such abuses were not new to Xinjiang, or to China for that matter. But the presence of increasingly rapacious Chinese officials provided fuel for unrest, and even a relatively minor incident could have unanticipated results. Having been in power for barely three years, Jin created just such an incident when he decided to abolish the traditional prerogatives of the prince of Komul (known to the Chinese as the prince of Hami) and to place the area under provincial control.

The death of the elderly prince in 1930 offered Jin the opportunity he sought to put an end to the small princedom. When the prince's young heir journeyed to Urumqi in order to protest, he was detained. While the prince's family had been neither popular nor fair, the new Chinese administration instituted by Jin was not an improvement, and Hami revolted. The movement escalated into a widespread movement to throw off Chinese rule and, in 1933, to establish a secessionist state, the East Turkestan Republic.

Jin had not expected vigorous opposition to his intervention in Hami. He was, after all, eliminating a ruler who still exercised old prerogatives such as corvée labor and capricious taxation of local residents. But his action not only aroused the animosity of Hami's residents: He also managed to alienate the contingent of "White" Russian troops, who had joined provincial forces under Governor Yang and were a staple of the local military. The leader of this group, the self-styled Colonel Papingut, led an insurrection in Urumqi against Jin in the spring of 1933, adding to the chaos already spreading as a result of the Hami revolt. In the midst of the crisis he had precipitated, Jin chose to flee, and his abrupt departure left a vacuum into which stepped the region's next Chinese warlord, General Sheng Shicai.

Sheng quickly came to an understanding with the Russian force, which agreed to support him. His military clout was further bolstered by additional Chinese troops, who had reached the border at Tacheng in January 1933, via the USSR. These men had been stationed in Manchuria; when the Japanese invaded in 1931, they had been forced to retreat into Soviet territory—southern Siberia—where they were detained. They were finally given permission to travel through the USSR for repatriation to China in Xinjiang. Traveling with their families, this force (known in PRC sources as the Northeast Volunteer Army) possibly included as many as 20,000 people, of which perhaps one-fifth were soldiers.[16] These newly arrived troops, plus the Russians and regular Han Chinese provincial forces, constituted the basis of Sheng's military strength, which, augmented by Soviet military support on several occasions, gave him control of Xinjiang for the next decade.

Sheng did not take the title of governor; rather, he resurrected the old title of military governor (*duban*) before finally taking the title of chairman (which replaced the earlier title of governor) in 1940. Regardless of his title, however, from 1933 to 1944 Sheng was the dominant figure in the government, and his policy toward the Kazaks, implemented with persistence and considerable success, directly contributed to great deterioration in Han-Kazak relations, leading to the Kazaks' involvement in the region's 1944 sucessionist movement.

Like Yang before him, Sheng first had to contend with warring factions in the province; but unlike Yang, Sheng faced Muslim armies rather than Han Chinese. As a result of Jin's actions in Hami, a Hui army unit from neighboring Gansu had entered eastern Xinjiang at the request of a delegation from Hami.[17] While this army posed a threat to the east, Sheng was soon faced with a second military threat in the south, where Uyghur leaders founded the Kashgar-based East Turkestan Republic in 1933. Although Sheng's army numbered an estimated 20,000 men in 1933, including well-trained, well-disciplined Russian troops, he now faced the possibility of a two-front war. Even more alarming was the threat of a united Muslim insurgency should the Komul group join forces with the new republic in Kashgar. With no possibility of assistance from China's central government, Sheng turned to the USSR. Support from Soviet military units enabled him to defeat the Muslim forces, executing captured leaders and driving others out of Xinjiang. By 1935 Sheng had restored order, and the reins of government were firmly in his hands.

Officially, Sheng's government espoused broadly democratic principles—in keeping with his public stance as part of the Chinese republic under the GMD and Chiang Kaishek. He first announced an "eight point policy," to be implemented through his "six great policies." Among other reforms, the latter called for the equality of all nationalities and freedom of religion; government relief for rural areas; financial, judicial, and administrative reforms; and clean government. Also in keeping with GMD policy, Sheng announced that his government was both anti-imperialist and pro-Soviet.[18]

As a first step toward ensuring the equality of all nationalities, it was necessary to identify clearly those groups who now qualified as "nationalities." Sheng recognized fourteen groups, which he identified as follows: Uyghur, Taranchi, Kazak, Kirghiz, Uzbek, Tatar, Tajik, Manchu, Xibo, Solon, Han, Hui, Mongol, and Russian. As discussed in Chapter 1, the name "Uyghur" referred to the sedentary Turkic population of the oases. Sheng was clearly following the Soviet example in the use of this ethnonym, which had been adopted in the USSR as a designation for Turkic-Muslims from Chinese Turkestan at their request.[19]

Sheng encouraged people to use only these names for self-identification through various means. First, he announced that there would be representatives of each nation in the provincial legislature to ensure a "voice" for each group. This was certainly a new development in the history of Chinese rule in the northwest; at the same time, it also meant that the Uyghurs, who constituted some 75 percent of the population, would now share power in the government with representatives of thirteen other groups—some of whom had only a few thousand members. Each nation would now compete with the others for a share of resources and political influence. This divide-and-rule policy had been used effectively throughout China's imperial past, when *yi yi zhi yi* was one of the standard tactics used by imperial China to manage the "barbarians" of the north, pitting them against each other as a way of both weakening them and deflecting attacks on China. Nonetheless, this promise of local participation in government may have contributed to the restoration of order upon the defeat of divided Muslim forces.

To give his new policies credibility, Sheng also announced the establishment of cultural associations for each of the fourteen nationalities. These officially sanctioned organizations gained members in the 1930s. The Uyghur Cultural Association, in particular, attracted a large, active membership. It offered its members a forum for the discussion of Turkic culture and, increasingly, for the dissemination of nationalist ideas. By the 1940s these cultural associations had become a base for strongly nationalistic Turkic groups.

Further, Sheng strengthened a sense of separate identities for Muslim groups by encouraging the publication of newspapers in various "national" languages as well as in Chinese, something Governor Yang had never allowed. Altogether, newspapers were published under Sheng in seven different languages, including Kazak.[20]

From the time of their creation until after 1950, the national cultural associations and the Turkic language publications were a problem for the provincial authorities, contributing to the evolution of strong national identities and to the idea that each nation was potentially the basis for a future independent state. Despite high illiteracy rates among some of the nationalities in the region, the newspapers reinforced the idea of national languages and served in the 1930s and 1940s to reinforce a growing national identity among some of the newly recognized "nationalities."[21]

Sheng's growing relationship with the USSR meant greater Soviet aid in exploiting natural resources. The Altay gold mines operated under the direction of Soviet engineers, as did oil wells at Wusu and Dushanzi. Of greater impact locally, however, was the expansion of trade with the USSR, which boosted the income of northwestern groups like the Kazaks.

From the Soviet side, trade was handled through the Soviet-Xinjiang Trade Agency, known locally as Sovinstorg, which opened branches in eight cities in Xinjiang in 1926. Despite Governor Yang's assassination in 1928, trade had continued to grow, so that by the early 1930s 82.5 percent of all Xinjiang's foreign trade was with the USSR. The most important export continued to be livestock and related products, which, by 1930–1933 accounted for 79–93 percent of all exports. Even oases in eastern Xinjiang like Turpan sold local products to the USSR. From Turpan to the nearest Chinese railhead in what is now Inner Mongolia was a journey of over 1,000 miles; once there, Turpan cotton still had to reach textile mills on the Chinese coast, where it competed with cotton imported from the United States and elsewhere. In 1930, the Turksib railway was completed, providing a rail connection that stimulated trade within Soviet Central Asia as well as increasing the market for Xinjiang products. As Table 3.2 shows, although trade dropped in 1931 and declined precipitously from 1933 to 1935 due to ongoing political and military turmoil in Xinjiang, once Sheng gained control, trade with the USSR again expanded rapidly. The main exports from Xinjiang continued to be animals, and the most valuable import from the Soviet Union remained cotton cloth.

Estimates on the number of animals in Xinjiang during the 1930s are inexact. Provincial figures for 1932 included 10 million sheep, 1.5 million horned cattle, 700,000 horses, 200,000 donkeys, and 90,000 camels.[22] In 1943, the province reported increases in the number of

Table 3.2

Xinjiang-Soviet Trade, 1929–1941

Year	Xinjiang Imports	Xinjiang Exports	Total Value
1929	1,643.5	1,639.6	3,283.1
1930	1,603.3	1,602.7	3,206.0
1931	1,021.2	1,394.5	2,415.7
1932	1,230.5	1,569.8	2,800.4
1933	1,882.2	1,085.6	2,967.8
1934	473.0	594.5	1,067.5
1935	604.9	455.0	1,059.9
1936	3,614.5	2,567.1	6,181.6
1937	3,475.3	2,577.4	6,052.7
1938	4,338.1	3,519.7	7,857.8
1939	3,310.7	4,170.0	7,480.7
1940	—	4,710.0	—
1941	4,709.7	4,370.0	9,079.7

Source: Li Sheng, *Xinjiang dui Su (E) maoyi shi 1600–1900* (1994), 409 and 479.
Note: Figures are given in units of 10,000 roubles.

sheep and goats for a total of 11,720,000, and of horses for a total of 870,000; figures for other kinds of animals were little changed from 1932.[23] By 1946, totals in all categories had risen. As taxes were levied on Kazaks according to the number of animals they owned, it is unlikely that correct numbers were reported; nonetheless, the above figures remain our best source for estimating the animal population during this period.

The demand for Xinjiang livestock was, in part, a result of the growth of new towns and cities in Soviet Central Asia, as suggested by Lattimore.[24] As more land was put into cotton, livestock pasturage decreased; urbanization and industrialization also contributed to the demand for Xinjiang livestock. Kazak resistance to Soviet attempts at collectivizing of their herds also reduced the numbers of animals, another factor in creating the strong demand for Xinjiang livestock. In return, Xinjiang imported Soviet manufactured goods, including cotton cloth, everyday kitchen utensils, crockery, glass, and electrical equipment. The USSR was also the major source of matches throughout the republican period.[25]

Sheng personally profited from Soviet-Xinjiang trade. Not only did he help establish the region's Provincial Commercial Bank, which issued a convertible currency, but in 1942 he also set up the Provincial

Trading Company, which Lattimore identified as Sheng's personal trading agent. Initially, it controlled 28 percent of Kashgar's trade, less than the percentage controlled by the single biggest Uyghur firm, Ittifat Sherket.[26]

In 1942 the Provincial Trading Company was given a monopoly on all trade with the USSR. It had the right to purchase local goods at prices set by the government, and it sold wool, livestock, cotton, and furs to Sovinstorg at great profit to Sheng and those involved in the company. Further, payment for local raw materials had been in Soviet manufactured goods, but in 1943, Sheng began paying partly in goods and partly in provincial-issued currency. The corruption of this and other related practices was so resented and harmful to the local business community that the company was liquidated in 1946. Despite the corruption, Soviet-Xinjiang trade remained vital to the people of Xinjiang, and many Kazaks enjoyed a relatively higher standard of living because of the demand for animal products in the USSR. Disruption in the market in the last years of Sheng's regime depressed nomads' income and most probably contributed to their willingness to join the 1944 rebellion against Chinese authority. As tables 3.3 and 3.4 suggest, a stable trading relationship with the USSR had become important to the nomadic economy by the 1940s. Nomadic nationalities owned an estimated two-thirds of Xinjiang livestock. The Kazak were therefore a key element of Xinjiang's economy during this period. Sheng sought to control this sector of the economy by controlling the nomads, but his aggressive policy led instead to their increased resistance.

Sources documenting both fragmented and organized Kazak resistance include both Chinese and Turkish accounts that, despite disagreement on some points, agree that such resistance became widespread in the early 1930s. A Kazak history of this period details a 1933 congress of Kazak leaders from all over Xinjiang that met at Koysu, in the Altay, to discuss how best to oppose Sheng's government. Influential leaders like Zayif Taiji, Ahid Haji, and Halil Taiji were among those calling for widespread resistance.[27] Kazak sources record that this meeting was reported by spies to the Chinese, who detained Ahid Haji and Halil Taiji not long after. Chinese troops then perpetrated what the Kazaks call *namys,* or affronts to national honor, by burning mosques, religious schools, and books in the town of Fuyun in northern Xinjiang.[28]

Table 3.3

Xinjiang Exports to the USSR, 1942–1945

	1942	1943	1944	1945
Wool	4,864	811	157	2,089
Cattle (head)	18,100	500	18,300	4,400
Sheep/Goats (head)	481,000	2,500	469,000	315,000
Horses (head)	50,000	2,200	19,000	25,500
Large hides (piece)	49,800	540	1,100	5,100
Small hides (piece)	1,548,000	12,700	7,300	118,000

Source: M.I. Sladovski, *Istorija torgovo-ekonomiceski otnosenij SSSR s Kitaem* [History of Trade and Economic Relations between the USSR and China] (1977), 158. Also in Li, Sheng, *Xinjiang dui Su (E) maoyi shi, 1600–1900* (1994), p. 521.

Table 3.4

Xinjiang Exports to the USSR, 1946–1949

	1946	1947	1948	1949
Wool	1,267	1,697	1,061	1,166
Cattle (head)	48,200	21,300	34,700	35,200
Sheep/Goats (head)	334,900	399,900	344,500	319,300
Small hides (piece)	520,000	495,000	379,000	412,000
Large hides (piece)	106,000	63,000	25,000	23,000
Intestines	516,000	829,000	642,000	631,000

Source: Sladovski, 158.

Chinese sources cast this history in a different light. They refer to Kazak plots to "foment chaos" in northern Xinjiang, naming men like the Kazak leader Sharif Han as among the organizers.[29] The many Kazak raids on Chinese and Uyghur settlements that continued through the 1930s were no doubt partly motivated by calls for resistance, entailing a degree of chaos in nomad areas, marked by raids on Chinese settlements and military posts. Increases in this kind of activity led to Chinese reprisals. At the same time, Sheng began a campaign to systematically disarm the Kazaks.

Kazak raids were not only an obstacle to peace in the region; in Sheng's view, this activity threatened his growing relationship with the

USSR and the important trade developing between his province and the Soviets. Sheng, therefore, began a series of "pacification" campaigns against the Kazaks in the mid-1930s. These were simultaneously reprisals for Kazak raids and part of his plan to disarm them or force them out of Xinjiang. Sheng used a network of spies and informers as part of his campaign. Further, highly respected, elderly Kazak leaders were kidnapped and used as hostages to force Kazaks to give up their arms and to leave their strongholds. As a result of these tactics, in the mid-1930s thousands of Kazaks abandoned pastures in northern Xinjiang and in the Tian Shan. Some moved into the Barkol area, but others were forced to move out of the region altogether. Kazaks entered western Gansu and also sought new pastures in the area of Qinghai's Ghoz Lake (Goz Kol), seeking to escape harassment from Sheng's troops. One group of some 4,000 Kazaks continued moving south, eventually making their way to India.

While Sheng's attempts to pacify the Kazaks forced some to flee, it also stiffened Kazak resistance to Sheng and his government. The most nationalistic of the new generation of Xinjiang Kazaks called for the establishment of a separate Kazak state in northern Xinjiang. Some were drawn to Uyghur nationalists who considered all the people of Xinjiang to be East Turkestani, rather than Uyghur, Kazak, or Kirghiz, and who called on all Muslims to rise against the "oppressor Chinese" in Xinjiang.[30] Others chose to launch their own local resistance movements. Initially, some groups sought only to retain their weapons and their traditional rights to pastures in northern Xinjiang. But as Sheng's onslaught against them continued, the numbers as well as the scale of activities against Sheng expanded.

In 1939–1940, Chinese troops stepped up their actions against Kazak strongholds. That winter, Chinese troops attacked the mosque of the arrested religious leader Ahid Haji in Sartogay. A demonstration against this attack was organized by two young Kazak leaders, Iris Han and Esim Han, in February 1940. When the Chinese authorities in the town moved to arrest them, the Kazaks fired on the Chinese and then fled.

One of the leaders around whom young Kazaks gathered that winter was Osman Batur. While he did not lead the majority of the region's Kazak population in the 1940s, an account of his activities during this last decade of republican rule in Xinjiang illustrates the complexity of the situation facing the Kazaks, divided between those allied to the

East Turkestan Republic of 1944–1949 and those choosing to follow leaders like Osman.

Osman was born in Russian territory, but he and his family crossed into China when Osman was still a child. A Kerey Kazak of the Molqi lineage, his name is linked to that of an earlier Kazak batur from the same line, Boke Batur, who had fought against the Qing for most of his life and was executed by the Chinese in Tibet in 1903.[31] Osman was married in 1918 or 1919 to Kaini, and the first of his sons, Serziman, was born in the Altay Mountains in 1920. By his own account, Osman's resistance to Sheng Shicai began in 1940—the same year in which Chinese reprisals against Kazaks in northern Xinjiang were intensified at places like Sartogay, as mentioned above.[32] According to Kazak accounts, in the winter of 1940, Sheng's troops rode into the camp of Osman's father, Islam Bay, demanding that all the men hand over their weapons. Osman alone reportedly refused, saying that if the Kazaks gave up their arms today they would give up their lives tomorrow. Taking his weapons, he and his eldest son then disappeared into the mountains.[33]

In March 1940, Osman was reportedly involved in a battle with Chinese troops at Baytik Bogdo, a mountainous area known to the Chinese as Beida Shan, on the present-day Chinese Mongolian border. Osman fought under the command of the Kazak leader, Nogabay, who like Osman had refused to give up his weapons. Nogabay had previously led attacks on Chinese border outposts, police stations, and Russian-operated mines. This time, Nogabay was killed in battle. His son, Iris Han, was elected to succeed his father, and Osman was elected second in command.[34] Iris Han and Osman fought Sheng's troops again in April. Kazak sources report that this time they were victorious, defeating a combined force of 8,000 Chinese and Russians, plus 200 soldiers from Mongolia—a victory not corroborated by other sources. Whether as a result of this encounter or not, Sheng decided to negotiate with the Kazaks in the spring of 1940. As conditions for peace, Iris Han demanded the release of political prisoners, the appointment of a Kazak as governor (district officer) of Altay, a prohibition of Russians working Altay gold mines, and an end to harassment and detention of Kazaks.

Negotiations succeeded, and an agreement was signed in July 1940. Osman, however, refused to be a party to any kind of settlement with Sheng. He and his followers left Iris Han, determined to continue fighting.

Sheng did, in fact, appoint a Kazak governor. He chose a pro-GMD Kazak leader, Janimhan, for this post. But at the same time, he also demanded an *amanat,* or hostage, ultimately detaining Janimhan's sons and some of his friends as a guarantee of Janimhan's support.[35]

In 1940, Sheng had other reasons to reach an understanding with the Kazaks. In that year, he had also signed a formal agreement with the USSR granting the Soviet Union extensive privileges in Xinjiang, including the right to prospect for and to exploit tin deposits. It was this provision that gave the contract the name of the Tin Mines Agreement.[36] The same agreement also allowed the USSR to build roads and to establish a communications network in northern Xinjiang, cutting through territory used for grazing by the Kazaks. Sheng also agreed that local residents in areas earmarked for Soviet exploitation would be moved.[37] The agreement, kept secret at the time, was another reason to increase efforts at pacifying the Kazaks, while at the same time maneuvering for their greater recognition of the government's authority.

Having rejected the agreement, Osman and his followers expanded their movement against the provincial authorities. By the end of 1940, Iris Han had died of "plague," and Esim Han had been killed fighting the Chinese, leaving Osman as the principal Kazak resistance leader in the north.

By 1942, Osman had an estimated following of 10,000 people. He led his men into battle against the Chinese repeatedly in that year, but his success was limited by a severe shortage of weapons. Sheng had collected so many guns from Kazak camps that when new recruits joined Osman they often brought only a few, antiquated weapons—and even these had to shared.[38] Osman himself told Doak Barnett, one of the few Americans to interview Osman in the late 1940s, that he negotiated to receive guns from Mongolia. Harassed by Sheng's troops in the winter of 1941–1942, Osman moved across the Chinese border into Mongolian territory, north of Ashan at Tayingol.[39] Here he reportedly met with Mongol representatives who promised whatever kind of support he needed to fight the Chinese, in exchange for a series of promises: Osman would send three of his men to Mongolia for education—his son, his brother, and a White Russian colleague; Osman would control his people, prohibiting them from crossing into Mongolian territory; Osman would accept the services of Mongolian advisors and 200 troops; and, finally, once he succeeded in taking northern Xinjiang, Osman would allow Mongolia to station men in

Qinghe and Fuyun. In return, Osman would be recognized as the governor of Altay as soon as he took control of the Ashan area. Religious freedom would be guaranteed, and there would be no communist propaganda. No Kazaks would be arrested, and Osman would receive whatever he needed to pursue his struggle against the Chinese.[40]

In the spring of 1942, the situation in Xinjiang changed abruptly. While Sheng had remained close to the USSR, he had also become increasingly wary of this alliance, distrustful of Soviet interest in Xinjiang and of his own military and government officials. Reassessing his position, he decided to abandon his Soviet alliance and realign with the Chiang government.

There were two immediate ramifications: First, the "private" Sheng-USSR agreements were abrogated; and, second, Sheng's previous welcome to members of the Chinese Communist Party was reversed. In April 1942, he detained all known CCP members and sympathizers, including Mao's brother, Mao Zemin, and several other high-ranking Chinese communists working in the provincial government. The most important figures were eventually executed, including Mao Zemin.[41]

This turnabout by Sheng threatened more than the Soviet political position; it was also a threat to the Soviet wartime economy, as livestock from Xinjiang had made an important contribution to Soviet food resources. In 1942, the new situation in Xinjiang meant that it was now in the Soviets' interest to supply men like Osman with weapons—as a counter to Sheng's change in allegiance and to forestall a possible decline in Xinjiang-Soviet trade. Although they could not approach Osman directly, the Soviets could use an intermediary like the Mongols to offer Osman the arms he desperately needed to oppose Sheng. Arming small guerrilla bands would not directly challenge the Chiang Kaishek government, with which the USSR still maintained official ties, but it would pose a challenge to the now-renegade Sheng. Further, the Soviets would have some control over Osman by controlling his source of weapons. If he grew to be a threat to Mongolian or Soviet interests, he could be eliminated—just as Soviet troops had eliminated Muslim units opposed to Sheng in the early 1930s.

For Osman's part, although he knew that his Mongol allies were aided by the Russians, his own need for weapons may have outweighed other considerations, and his decision to accept arms from this quarter was perhaps made easier because the Mongols, too, were struggling to oust the Chinese from their territory.

Sheng's 1942 reversal of allegiance also meant a drastic change in Soviet-Xinjiang trade patterns. The official figures from the Soviet side indicate that during 1942–1943 trade dropped drastically. The group most hurt by this change was the Kazaks: The amount of wool sold to the USSR dropped from 4,864 tons in 1942 to only 811 tons in 1943; likewise, the number of sheep and goats fell from 481,000 head to only 2,500 head. As tables 3.3 and 3.4 show, all major exports dropped in these years. Deprived of important sources of income, Kazaks correctly blamed Sheng. The incidence of Kazak attacks on government posts and garrisons dramatically increased in the summers of 1942 and 1943.

In September, Osman was wounded in a battle with Sheng's troops and withdrew to a camp near the Mongolian border.[42] He was in this camp when Sheng's troops attacked him. In Osman's defense, on March 12–13, 1944, Mongol planes retaliated and attacked the Chinese. According to Soviet sources, the Chinese were totally to blame for this border incident. These sources reported that the Xinjiang provincial government was forcing Kazaks to move to the south and that some of them, in defiance of this order, had fled into the Mongolian border area. Chinese planes, they said, had pursued the Kazaks, violating Mongol airspace. Because the 1936 mutual aid pact between Mongolia and the USSR obliged the Soviets to come to the aid of Mongolia, it had done so, driving the Chinese planes away and counterattacking.[43] For their part, the Chinese lodged an official protest over this border incursion by the Soviet Union. The incident remained unresolved and was soon to be repeated as Osman took advantage of the protection afforded him by the proximity of the Mongolian border.[44]

Foreign officials stationed in the region noted that Kazak unrest became widespread in 1943–1944. In the winter of 1944, Sheng contributed further to existing tensions by issuing an order requisitioning horses. A total of 10,000 horses were to be "donated" by the people of Xinjiang to the war effort, the number of animals being apportioned among the ten districts of the province.[45] Money was accepted in lieu of horses, fixed at a price of 750 Xinjiang dollars, a price far above the market value.[46]

Sheng's intention in issuing such an order may have been to please the Guomindang with a sizable contribution of horses to the war effort; but given the logistical problems of delivering such a number of animals to China proper, another motive seems more likely: to increase the coffers of the provincial government and its chief. Certainly the order netted far more money than horses. Thus, the requisition appears to have been a ploy to accumulate capital, possibly to pave the way for Sheng's reentrance into the Guomindang fold.[47]

Whatever the purpose in issuing a requisition order, it was certain to cause opposition. By the end of March 1944, the *Xinjiang ribao,* published in Urumqi, announced that the Ashan District, the heart of the Kazak Altay region, had donated a total of one hundred horses. Of these, the Kazak Cultural Society gave twenty animals, while officials of other Kazak groups gave another twenty.[48] No further reports of contributions from the Altay appeared in the local press, suggesting that this small number was the most the government could squeeze from one of the major horse-breeding areas in the region.

In the spring and summer of 1944, Chinese efforts at "bandit suppression" increased throughout the northern districts of Xinjiang in response to an ever-increasing number of raids, which were attributed to the Kazak. In July 1944, Kazaks attacked the town of Jimunai, near the Sino-Soviet border. According to Chinese sources, the Kazaks received weapons to use in this attack from Soviet trucks that had been driven up to the frontier.[49] The Kazaks involved in this attack were not Osman's people. Instead, they were among the Kazak groups disaffected by Sheng's break with the USSR, an event that, as noted earlier, had severely hampered trade between Xinjiang and the Soviet Union. But Osman, too, continued to oppose Sheng, defeating Chinese forces in battles at Sagan and Dontu, in the summer of 1944. When reinforcements were sent out to attack him, Osman once again retreated, this time moving into the Barkol area, northwest of the oasis town of Hami in the late summer or early autumn of 1944.[50]

In September 1944, negotiations between the GMD and Sheng resulted in Sheng's departure for the wartime capital of Chongqing. For the first time since 1912, the GMD had the opportunity to control directly the far northwest.

**Nationalist Rule in Xinjiang and the
East Turkestan Republic**

Chiang Kaishek appointed Wu Zhongxin to replace Sheng as the top official in Xinjiang. Before Governor Wu arrived, in October 1944, Kazaks from Barkol raided the provincial capital itself. When this raiding party withdrew, Chinese troops were sent out to the towns of Qiande and Fugang to reinforce guard posts there. No pursuit of the Kazaks followed, however, and no additional patrols were organized to protect the capital from such bold "bandits."[51] By the time the new governor made his appearance in Urumqi at the end of October, he faced a more serious threat than Kazak raids. In early November, the region was torn by the upheavals of a new separatist movement based at Yining in the Ili Valley. There, on November 12, 1944, a new East Turkestan Republic was established under President Ali Han Tore, an Uzbek religious scholar with a strong local following. Other key leaders who emerged in the winter of 1944–1945 included two Uyghurs, Ahmetjan Kasimi and Abdul Kerim Abbas, and a Kirghiz military leader, Ishak Han Mura Haji. They led a combined movement of Uyghurs, Kazaks, White Russians, Kirghiz, Xibo, and Hui.

With weapons purchased from the USSR, the army of the new republic quickly defeated Chinese forces in the towns of the Ili Valley. Victorious, the Ili army drove north and east, defeating Chinese troops and forcing civilians to flee; some refugees crossed the border into the USSR for protection, while others streamed out of the border area toward the safety of the provincial capital.

In response, the new governor organized a special committee for "pacification" in November 1944, under the Commission for Civil Affairs and with branches in the districts of Altay, Ili, and Tacheng (Tarbagatay).[52] In December, Wu announced that one of the new commissioners was to be Alin Wang, a member of the hereditary Kazak nobility who had been jailed by Sheng and was now being released.[53] Wang's official title was Vice Administrative Supervisor of the Altay.[54] His first assignment was to pacify the Kazaks who had raided the provincial capital in October, by persuading them to support the government. He was to "promote trust" among the Kazaks and to convey Governor Wu's pledge of religious freedom.[55] By that winter, however, fighting erupted in the northern area of the region between government forces and the Kazaks. In January 1945, as the fighting in the Ili area began to spill out of the valley, Osman was besieging two Chinese guard posts in northeastern Xinjiang. Osman cut supply routes to the area in an effort to prevent any of his beleaguered enemies from receiving aid or escaping. But in March, the desperate Chinese forces broke the siege and fled. Osman was, nonetheless, credited with a victory by Kazaks for freeing the area from Chinese rule.[56]

According to Chinese sources, Alin Wang had been sent up to the Altay area in February 1945, during Osman's siege of the Chinese guard posts. His mission was clearly unsuccessful, and he returned to the provincial capital some months later having been unable to dissuade Kazaks from joining the East Turkestan Republic. Although his overall mission failed, he met with Osman at least once during his visit, and may have planted the seeds of Osman's later defection to the GMD side.[57]

In May 1945, East Turkestani forces intensified their attacks. The Ashan District's capital, Chenghua (Sharasume), was attacked by men with machine guns and mortars. Chinese defenders identified Osman and his men among the attacking force. It was later reported that the tactics used in this battle were quite different from the usual nomad battle plan, suggesting outside leadership.[58] However, even if facing externally led forces, the Chinese at Chenghua did not readily capitulate. They held out through the summer. Again according to Chinese sources, Mongolian and Soviet reinforcements aided the rebels in midsummer. On August 11 and 13, the Chinese commander begged for air support against these attacks, but the provincial authorities were slow to react. Without support, the Chinese abandoned the city during the first week of September 1945. The city was occupied by Osman and representatives of the East Turkestan Republic.[59]

By the autumn of 1945, Osman had allied himself to the Ili-based republic. He was made East Turkestan's governor in the Altay area, with his capital at Chenghua, and his men became a part of the extensive Kazak cavalry already allied to the new nation. This victory gave the republic control of three of Xinjiang's ten districts. Their combined territory amounted to 20 percent of the province and a total of 16–20 percent of the total population. Over half the population of the three districts was Kazak.

Further south, East Turkestani forces had reached the bank of the Manas River, bringing them to within ninety kilometers of the provincial capital. In panic, Chinese officials sent their families to Hami, the first step in their evacuation from Xinjiang. It appeared that the city would fall to the approaching forces.

Instead, a cease-fire was arranged in the middle of the month through the mediation of the USSR. The East Turkestani army remained on the western bank of the Manas River, which became the de facto border between the three districts controlled by the republic and the rest of the region. Peace talks began between East Turkestani representatives and the GMD, and in January 1946 a settlement was made between the two sides, paving the way for a formal peace agreement, which was signed on June 6, 1946, in Urumqi. That July, a new provisional government formed, combining Nationalist-GMD appointees with representatives of East Turkestan's ethnically mixed leadership. The new government was to oversee implementation of the peace agreement, leading to autonomy for Xinjiang's Muslims. The three districts would remain a part of China, to be reincorporated into the provincial administration.

For his part in the fighting, Osman was among those awarded a government post. On August 20, 1946, the main Chinese language newspaper in Urumqi announced his appointment as the new district officer of Ashan, which included the Altay areas he had been seeking to preserve for his people.

Other Kazaks were also named to posts in the new government. Unlike Osman, who remained in the Altay area, these appointees arrived to take up their new posts in Urumqi. Of greatest importance to Osman was Janimhan, the former governor of the Ashan District under Sheng, who became the new minister of finance in August 1946. Also appointed was Salis Remek, one of two new deputy secretaries-general under GMD appointee Liu Mengchun. Unlike Osman, both of these men were appointees of the Chinese provincial government rather than of the Ili group.

Osman was evidently very pleased with this appointment. In a letter to the Xinjiang garrison commander, Song Xilian, Osman vowed to uphold Sun Yatsen's Three Principles of the People, to attack any Mongols who dared enter the Beida Shan, and to protect all of Ashan's people.[60] Osman also reportedly contacted General Zhang Zhizhong, the peace negotiator who had replaced Governor Wu Zhongxin as the regional chairman, and who now led the new coalition provincial government.

Further, Chinese sources assert that in a statement written at his direction, Osman announced that he could no longer support the East Turkestani republican movement. He explained that while he had initially supported the republic, its leaders had cheated the people of Xinjiang by allying East Turkestan to the USSR. As he remained adamantly anti-Soviet, Osman could no longer give them his support.[61]

There is no document available to corroborate this, and Osman later offered a different account of his decision to end support for the East Turkestan Republic in 1946. In an interview with journalist Ian Morrison in 1948, Osman said that he had cooperated with the republic until April 1946, after which time he went to Beida Shan. The republic, he said, had insisted that Osman attend a meeting in Ili, at which time they demanded that he transfer control of his people to the Ili government and also allow East Turkestani officials to take over the garrison in the Altay capital. He had other grievances as well: He mentioned that Kazak women had been taken away to Ili, angering his people; that the East Turkestan Republic was allowing the Soviets to continue their mining operations in the Altay; and that the East Turkestani government had taken 28,000 ounces of gold that had been the property of the Altay government. All of these appear to have figured in his decision to *touming*, to change allegiance, to the GMD rather than to continue as an ally of East Turkestan. Only after making these varied points did Osman give what he called his real reasons for turning against the new republic. First, he said that communism was hostile to religion, implying that East Turkestan was now under Soviet control; second, he said that the Ili government was encroaching on Chinese national territory, a rather incongruous statement considering he had fought for six years against a man who was ostensibly the representative of the Chinese; and third, he said that the Kazak people would get a "better deal" from the Chinese than from the Russians.[62] It remains difficult to assess Osman's true motives in switching his allegiance. Nevertheless, while interviews and other sources attribute Osman's defection to a variety of reasons— ranging from financial gain to patriotic feelings for China—Osman's subsequent actions place him squarely in the GMD camp.

Osman's defection from the East Turkestan Republic did not have an immediate impact on the Ili-based movement, which had maintained its authority in the three districts despite the peace agreement signed by its representatives. However, criticism quickly emerged over Osman's public denunciation of the republic and its goals. Rumors circulated suggesting that Osman's Kazaks had been bribed to join the Chinese and that they were serving as mercenaries for the Chinese military. There is indirect proof that Osman did, in fact, receive large payments that may have influenced his decision to desert the East Turkestani cause. The new provincial minister of finance, Janimhan, was a Kazak from the Altay area, like Osman. In 1946, Janimhan was also appointed the head of the election committee that was to supervise elections in the Ashan district. As part of the 1946 peace agreement, elections were to be held in each district, and district election committees were the first step in the process. Appointed to serve with Janimhan were Osman and his assistant, Latif.[63] The number of meetings or the types of communication between Janimhan and Osman in 1946 is unclear, but there were important financial dealings between the provincial government and the Altay government of which Osman was still the head. In July 1946, the new government in Urumqi allotted $40 million for the "relief of the three districts," a share of which was earmarked for Ashan.[64] In May 1947, a special allotment of money was made to Ashan alone; according to newspaper reports, a payment of $30 million was given to this area in recognition of the past bitter years.[65] Osman was still officially the district officer and would presumably have had access to these funds. Whether these were intended as "bribes" or payments for his services as a mercenary may never be known; but in the winter of 1946–1947, Osman clearly shifted away from the East Turkestan Republic and firmly allied himself and his people with the GMD.

Osman's change of allegiance meant that the region's Kazaks were now divided. As noted earlier, Osman and his people represented only a minority of the total Kazak population. Nonetheless, they played an important role in the political struggle that continued in Xinjiang; they soon joined military expeditions on behalf of the GMD, giving their small numbers a disproportionate impact on events.

During the winter of 1946–1947, the provisional coalition government in Urumqi was struggling to maintain at least a semblance of unity. The Ili members of the coalition awaited evidence that the reforms called for in the peace agreement would, in fact, be carried out. The Chinese uneasily noted that a new, defiant spirit seemed to be growing steadily among the local population, including the Uyghurs and Kazaks they had considered most supportive of an expanded and strengthened GMD role in Xinjiang. While the promised elections were held more or less on schedule, the Chinese were simultaneously increasing the number of Chinese troops in Xinjiang. By 1947, between 90,000 and 100,000 Han Chinese troops were stationed there— ten times the number of troops under Governor Yang.[66] The presence of so many troops quickly made itself felt. As it was impossible to supply them from China proper, they had to be fed and otherwise provisioned from the local economy. The strain on local resources was considerable. In February 1947, rioters took to the streets of the provincial capital, with Muslim groups demonstrating against the government one day and Chinese groups counterdemonstrating the next. After several days of violence, General Song Xilian, the highest-ranking Chinese officer present, ordered the army in to restore order. Zhang, who had been out of the province, quickly returned, but the coalition government he had built over the preceding seven months was clearly in trouble.

Anger toward the government directly involved the loyalties of the Xinjiang Kazaks. An important issue continued to be who would represent the Kazaks and who should hold government appointments to Kazak districts. As Osman was no longer in the East Turkestan camp, its supporters wanted him dismissed as Ashan district officer. When the provincial government refused, the republic rescinded its own appointment of Osman as the governor of Ashan and appointed as his replacement a loyal Kazak military leader, Delilhan.[67]

Early in the winter of 1947, troops from the still-extant East Turkestan Republic went against Osman, beginning a series of bloody battles. By April, Osman and his followers retreated, moving first to Kuerte in April 1947 and then once more to the Beida Shan on the Mongolian border, where they remained into the late spring of 1947.

Osman's adventures had already contributed to the tensions in the provincial government. That spring the coalition collapsed. Zhang had sought to repair the damage done to the GMD by the February riots by making a spring tour of the southern oases. At virtually every stop, he had been met with demands from the local population for the immediate removal of the Chinese troops who had arrived since Sheng's departure. In May, when a crowd in Kashgar nearly rioted during one of his speeches, Zhang cut his tour short and returned to the capital. That same month he resigned as chairman, and the GMD appointed a locally born Uyghur, Mesut Sabri, as the new chairman.

Mesut's long association with the GMD made him suspect in the eyes of East Turkestani members of government, and they immediately objected to his appointment, demanding that Zhang remain as chairman. When it was clear that their view on this matter—like on the appointment of Osman—was not going to be respected, these members withdrew, returning to Ili that spring.

Mesut's appointment was only the culmination of acts that were viewed by the East Turkestan Republic and its sympathizers as not in keeping with either the spirit or the actual terms of the peace agreement. One factor that clearly was a cause of much bitterness was the Chinese alliance with their former ally, Osman, who, it was believed, was being used by the Chinese to harass the three districts while the Chinese continued to build their military strength. In May 1947, newspapers in the three East Turkestani districts vehemently attacked Osman for his "treachery" against the fatherland, Turkestan. His crimes were listed as opposition to the peace agreement, destruction of public order and security, and cooperation with "criminals."[68] The latter included Salis, who was then serving as deputy secretary-general of the provincial government, and Hadewan, the wife of pro-GMD Alin Wang. A formidable person in her own right, Hadewan was the district officer of Urumqi, the only minority woman to hold a position of power in the entire province.

From May 1947 onwards, Osman strengthened his alliance with the Chinese Nationalists. In the early summer of 1947, Osman was involved in the Beida Shan incident, which occurred on the Sino-Mongolian border, where Osman had camped many times. The border incident briefly drew international attention, but it was insignificant in comparison with Osman's autumn 1947 assault on the Altay area in an attempt to take control of Chenghua and to resume his position as the head of the Ashan district. Leading some 2,000–3,000 men armed with Nationalist-supplied weapons, Osman took the towns of Chinghe and Fuyun before stopping to prepare for the onslaught on Chenghua. While the Nationalist-controlled press in Urumqi reported his victories and published flattering accounts of Osman as a loyal patriot, the East Turkestani forces prepared well for his arrival. By the middle of October, he was once more driven from the Altay area, for the last time.[69]

Osman's ignominious expulsion from the Altay area does not, however, mark the end of his activities in Xinjiang. Now nearly fifty years old and a veteran of many battles, he and his followers appeared willing to accept the largesse of the Chinese Nationalist government. In addition to supplying him with food and military supplies, the Chinese government announced in December 1947 that Osman's eldest son, Serziman, would serve as one of Xinjiang's delegates to the national assembly of China. Also appointed was a friend and fellow warrior of Osman, Hamza Uchar, as well as other Kazak allies and friends.[70]

By 1948, Chiang Kaishek's government was in an extremely precar-

ious position. Repeated military losses made the future of his government uncertain, and Xinjiang, like other parts of the country, now
awaited the final outcome.

Possibly in an attempt to garner last-minute local support for the
Guomindang, the unpopular Mesut was removed from office and replaced in early 1949 with Burhan Shahidi, a Tatar who had been serving as vice-chairman. It was to be Burhan who would preside over the
transfer of power in Xinjiang from the Guomindang to the CCP in
September 1949.

That summer, as the People's Liberation Army approached
Xinjiang's western border, the representatives of foreign powers in
Urumqi began leaving. The British alone chose not to abandon totally
their office in Xinjiang; their representative, George Fox-Holmes, was
thus present for the last days of GMD control in the region. The United
States consul, John Hall Paxton, left for India, leaving behind Doug
MacKiernan who, in September, burned consulate documents remain-
ing in the Urumqi office and handed over the office equipment to
Fox-Holmes.

Rather than attempting to cross into India, MacKiernan instead
headed for Osman's camp, taking with him anthropologist and OSS
agent Frank Bessac, who had chosen to leave China by the longest
possible route, via Xinjiang. The two men stayed with Osman during
the winter of 1949–1950, and when the snows began to melt in spring
of 1950, they began their journey out. With guides supplied by the
Kazaks and accompanied by several White Russians, they made their
way to Tibet. In a sudden attack by Tibetans, MacKiernan was shot
and killed, leaving a badly shaken Bessac to make his way on to India
alone with what remained of their party.[71]

While the two Americans were seeking Osman, the PLA had continued on its way to Xinjiang. In late September, Governor Burhan and
the local GMD military garrison commander, Tao Zhiyue, tele-
grammed their welcome to the new government, a process eased by the
defection of Zhang Zhizhong to the CCP in the summer of 1949. The
GMD troops stationed in seven of the region's ten districts guaranteed
a relatively peaceful transition as they were ordered to remain in place
until relieved by the PLA, the first contingents of which reached the
provincial capital in October. Burhan retained his position temporarily,
as the CCP extended its control over the region.

Prior to the PLA's arrival, secret negotiations began between the

CCP and the still extant East Turkestan Republic. Invited to Beijing for talks, four of the top ETR leaders died in a plane crash en route, robbing the ETR of its most able and charismatic leaders. In December, China's new government announced the incorporation of the ETR military into the PLA, bringing to an end the independence of Xinjiang's second East Turkestan Republic.

As the CCP moved to resolve any possible military threat from the three districts in the late summer of 1949, groups of Kazaks met to discuss what they should do. Some chose to move to remote Ghoz Kol (Goz Lake) in Qinghai, an old meeting place for Kazaks in times of crisis. From there, some groups decided to move on to Tibet and then to India. Remnants of these groups ultimately made their way to Turkey, forming the basis of today's Kazak community there.

Others, however, wanted to fight. Osman became the rallying point for many of these men, as well as for small numbers of White Russians who added to available firepower. Janimhan, the former finance minister, joined Osman, and other leaders sent their representatives to discuss the situation. After the PLA entered the region in October, communication became more difficult due both to their presence and to the harsh winter that descended.

The newly arrived PLA sent emissaries to the Kazaks, hoping to persuade them to support the new government, as Burhan and a handful of Kazaks in Urumqi had decided to do. Osman and the others refused these overtures, but by the end of the year, the Kazaks had to make a decision. In December, Ali Beg Hakim, a sometime colleague and friend of Osman's, decided he would leave Xinjiang, first heading for Ghoz Kol. He came to his decision after talking with the other leaders, most of whom now believed that resistance was futile. Osman and Janimhan came to the same conclusion and began the trek to Qinghai in spring of 1950. En route, they were attacked by units of the PLA and Janimhan was captured. Disheartened and carrying many wounded, Osman's group continued south.

In late 1950, Osman reached an area called Kanambal Mountain by the Kazaks, near Makai in Qinghai province. Kazaks who were there recall the poor condition of Osman's camp that winter. Rather than move in the winter weather, he decided to remain there until conditions improved. But the PLA troops successfully tracked him, and on February 15, 1951, they surrounded the camp and took Osman prisoner.

With great public fanfare, Osman was tried as a bandit and thief in the capital of Urumqi. Specifically, he was accused of killing 230 people and of being responsible for the deaths of a further 1,175, of all nationalities. He was also accused of stealing 340,000 animals and vast quantities of supplies and of destroying the homes of thousands of people. He was, according to the new government, a "scourge of peaceful society."[72]

Osman's alliance with the GMD and his protection and aid to Doug MacKiernan and Frank Bessac meant that he was also forced to confess to being an "imperialist armed spy," working for the American government. In a lengthy written confession, he wrote that he had been directed by MacKiernan since the 1947 Beida Shan incident and that together they had formed the "Anti-Communist, Anti-Soviet, and Anti-Three Districts Revolutionary Committee," for which Osman had gathered intelligence. MacKiernan, according to the confession, had remained in Xinjiang in order to continue to direct Osman's activities against the CCP. Osman was found guilty of all charges and executed in April 1951.

Osman's execution was intended as a warning to the remaining groups of Kazaks opposed to the imposition of a communist government in Xinjiang. Despite the warning, however, pockets of armed Kazaks and other Muslims continued resistance through 1954.

As detailed in the following chapter, the 1949 arrival of the PLA did not signal immediate, significant changes for the Kazaks as a group. Some sought an accommodation with the CCP, while others attempted simply to ignore the new authorities. Whatever tactic they chose to pursue, however, the Kazaks soon discovered that, unlike the previous, relatively inept regime, the new government was intent on revolutionary changes for all of Xinjiang's people. Within a decade, the impact of new policies, implemented by a government with the power to enforce them, would change their lives in ways no Chinese government had ever been able to do before.

4

CCP Minority Policy
and Its Implementation
in Xinjiang

Prior to 1949, the Chinese Communist Party appears to have given relatively little thought to how it would handle minority regions once it gained power. One result of this was that the PRC's minority policy evolved through several distinct phases after 1949—more reactive than ideological and more pragmatic than planned. As the following discussion illustrates, minority policy flowed along channels that allowed broad and then narrow interpretations of Marxist thought on the "national question," leaving uncertainty and distrust among peoples like the Kazaks by the 1990s.

Constitutions, Minority Rights, and Legal Status

The earliest written statement on the CCP's minority policy dates from the party platform of 1931. At that time, the CCP declared that non-Han Chinese areas of China would be allowed to secede or to federate with the Chinese state, according to the will of each group. This stand was theoretically in keeping with the ideas of Dr. Sun Yatsen, whose initially assimilationist stance on minority issues had evolved by 1923 into a pluralist position that included the possibility of self-determination for peoples like the Mongols and Tibetans. While the separate cultural identities of these two groups was clearly accepted by Dr. Sun, it is less clear as to whether he would have accorded the same recognition to other, less numerous minority groups. During the party's early decades, as the CCP presented itself as heir to the mantle of Dr. Sun, his acceptance of a China composed of five separate nations became a part of its doctrine, such as it was, on minority rights.

By 1938, however, party documents no longer referred to any such right; instead, the party's socialist revolution was to benefit all people equally, with all Chinese territory remaining an integral part of the state. It is possible that this change was in recognition of foreign powers' efforts at dividing the Chinese state; it may also have been a reaction to the Japanese occupation of Manchuria. What it does *not* appear to be is an extension of a particular theoretical, Marxist position.[1] Rather, this policy change was an *ad hoc* reaction to existing political realities.

After 1949, the first official statements on China's national minorities and their rights were in the Common Program, a wide-ranging document passed by the Chinese People's Political Consultative Conference of 1949.[2] Five articles of the Common Program are relevant to China's ethnic minorities. First, article 9 declared that no area of China may secede. Thus China, unlike its neighboring Soviet communist ally, decreed itself a unitary state, no part of which could choose separation from the whole. Second, article 50 stated that both Han chauvinism and "local" chauvinism should be opposed. This article was thus a recognition of the attitude of cultural superiority that marked Chinese regard for some minorities, an attitude that posed a potential obstacle to party work. But it was also recognition of repeated minority rebellion against the central Chinese government in the years of the republic. Third, article 51 called for the establishment of autonomous organs of government in areas entirely or largely inhabited by national minorities. Fourth, article 52 guaranteed equal rights for all nationalities in China and further stated that all Chinese citizens have freedom of religion and of culture, as well as the freedom to continue traditional practices. These same freedoms, plus a good many more, had been guaranteed to minorities like the Kazaks by preceding governments with little effect; likewise, while these assurances were doubtless welcome in some circles, the Common Program gave no indication how these personal freedoms would be guaranteed or what group or groups would provide redress if such freedoms were violated. Finally, article 53 stated that the central government would aid in the development of the national minority areas. Such aid had been promised during the republic, but in fact very little had been done. Development of the regional economy was certainly something local leadership in minority areas would favor; yet, government aid also implied a greater Chinese presence and, most likely, a greater Chinese control over local affairs.

Of the various plans and principles encompassed in these articles, the autonomous organs of government called for in article 51 were considered fundamental to China's solution of the "national question."[3] Although its rhetoric owed much to the Soviet model, the Common Program differed in fundamental ways from Soviet policy. Most importantly, it did not hold out the possibility of a minority territory seceding from China—a right retained in principle in the USSR. While no area was allowed to secede, the CCP did seek to deal more creatively with the complex ethnic mixture in some of its territory.

Despite the existence of the Common Program and its assurances for minorities, CCP activity in minority areas appears to have been less an outgrowth of the party's ideological positions than the result of pragmatic decisions made in the field. In several areas (in particular, Tibet, Xinjiang, and Inner Mongolia) the PLA was guided only by general pronouncements from Beijing leaders, who were simultaneously dealing with the massive challenge of reconstruction their victory had brought. The first order of business was simply to establish complete military domination of all regions of China; the second priority was the imposition of Communist Party control over all political and social institutions.[4]

The instrument for establishing the party's power was the PLA. Composed primarily of Han Chinese, the PLA was to occupy all areas and eliminate the Guomindang and any other enemies of the people's revolution. Available sources on the process by which the PLA inaugurated CCP rule in border and minority regions are scant; recent works that do include discussion of these early years generally gloss this period as the "peaceful liberation," a time in which the masses of the Chinese people "stood up," finally freeing themselves from oppressive GMD rule. The lack of detail available suggests—among other things—that policy was, indeed, an ad hoc response to conditions, rather than the result of a predetermined set of principles.

That there were still policy details to work out is also suggested by the fact that it was not until 1953 that specific details for the implementation of the autonomous governments called for in article 52 were announced, in a document entitled the "Program for Enforcement of National Regional Autonomy." According to this document, there were three different circumstances under which an area could claim autonomous status in China. First were the districts inhabited predominantly by one national minority; second were the districts where one minority constituted a numerical majority and that were also inhabited by several less populous groups; third were the districts inhabited by two or more minorities. In any of these circumstances, governments would be run "principally" by the national minorities themselves.

In fact, few areas qualified for the first designation. By 1958, four regional-level autonomous governments had been formed, each recognizing the predominance of a particular group. These were the Xinjiang-Uyghur, Ningxia, Inner Mongolia, and Guangxi-Zhuang Autonomous Regions. Tibet, which had the greatest concentration of one single minority, did not receive autonomous region status until 1965.

All five autonomous regions included other nationalities within their borders. As each national minority was entitled to representation in the regional government, power had to be divided among all minorities as well as the Han Chinese, themselves a minority in Tibet and Xinjiang in 1949. In Xinjiang, this initially meant a division of power among fourteen separate nationalities. However, by the 1990s, as a result of migration into the region, Xinjiang had members of fifty different nationalities, necessitating even further division of power. While most in-migration represented relatively small numbers of new arrivals and therefore had a limited impact, the great number of migrant Han Chinese radically changed the ethnic composition of most minority regions. Today, while Tibet and Xinjiang still have a single, numerically dominant non-Han majority (the Tibetans and the Uyghurs, respectively), the number of Han Chinese has risen so dramatically that they are now the second most numerous nationality, entitled to a proportionate role in local governments.

This phenomenon was begun by the forceful relocation of Han Chinese to border regions to hasten economic development there, but in the 1980s increasing numbers of Han Chinese migrated to these areas of their own accord, reflecting new economic freedom, which has included greater freedom of movement. Han in-migration has become a major issue in Xinjiang and other autonomous areas—a theme to which we return in chapters 6 and 7. The arrival of large numbers of Han has decreased minority representation in autonomous governments, for the requirement that all nationalities be represented in government still remains in force.

Lower-level autonomous governments were formed within the autonomous regions as well as in the ordinary provinces. Levels include the prefecture (*zhou*) and the county (*xian*); at these levels, too, power was apportioned among all minority groups; and as virtually all of these smaller units had at least several minority nationalities as well as Han Chinese, it was impossible for any single group to dominate any government.

Powers reserved for these autonomous governments were considerable. They could, within the limits of the Chinese constitution and legal code, organize local militia, develop local culture, use local languages as their official language, and control local finances. If such power had been fully utilized as outlined in official documents, national minorities would have controlled vast territories within the PRC. However, two factors made this impossible from the very beginning. First, as noted above, no autonomous area and therefore no autonomous government at any level was composed solely of one nationality. Even in counties where one nationality accounted for more than 50 percent of the local population, every minority had to be represented in the government—and, always, places had to be reserved for Han Chinese. As will be seen in the discussion of the Xinjiang's three Kazak autonomous areas in chapter 5, power was shared from the very beginning.

The second factor in limiting minority autonomy was the role of the PLA and the CCP in all the minority regions in the first decade of Communist rule. Both powerful institutions were virtually all Han Chinese. Very few minority cadres attained high rank in either organization. Those officials who had some minority connection—such as Deng Xiaoping and his Hakka background—ignored this connection, preferring to be only Han. The few exceptions were mainly Hui—Chinese Muslims whose Islamic faith had long been sacrificed to CCP atheism, and Mongols like Ulanhu, the sinified Mongol leader, who no longer spoke Mongolian. Other non-Han leaders of minority movements in the 1930s and 1940s were either co-opted or eliminated, as we have already seen in the cases of Burhan Shahidi and Osman Batur. Although local minority leaders were chosen as figureheads to lead autonomous governments, power remained in the hands of the Han leadership of the party and the military. As in preceding centuries, Han Chinese dominated all positions of real power. By 1957 there were eighty-seven autonomous districts, thirty-one autonomous prefectures (*zhou*) and fifty-four autonomous counties (*xian*), all creations of the Chinese-dominated CCP.

National minority rights were also included in the first Chinese constitution, in 1954. With nearly five years of practical experience in governing minority regions, the PRC now modified its early position with regard to minority rights and government structure in minority areas. In the first constitution, governments of national minority regions were to be composed of an "appropriate" number of national minority representatives, rather than "principally" of national minority peoples as called for in the Common Program.[5] This change was in recognition of the fact that there would be a need for Chinese leadership in national minority areas for some time to come if the social reform envisioned by the CCP was to be properly implemented. It was also now recognized that there were too few CCP cadres from among the national minorities—and those who were party members were too inexperienced to lead governmental or party organs in sensitive and still politically unstable border regions.

Succeeding Chinese constitutions, from 1954 to 1978, consistently referred briefly to five basic propositions that can be regarded as the basis of Chinese minority policy through 1978. These five propositions are as follows: (1) China is a multinational and unitary state, and no area may secede; (2) regional autonomy is the basic form of government for all areas inhabited by national minorities; (3) there is equality for all nationalities within China; (4) there is freedom to believe and not to believe in religion; (5) national minority peoples have the right to use their national languages in written and in spoken forms.

The 1982 constitution reaffirmed these five basic points, adding greater detail. In both the 1978 and 1982 constitutions, chapter 1, article 4 calls for equality for all nationalities and for the protection of such rights by the state. Each constitution also prohibits any discrimination against a single nationality, and the 1982 constitution adds the line that "any acts that undermine the unity of the nationalities or *instigate their secession are prohibited.*"[6]

Further, the 1982 constitution also provides more detail on the organs of government for national autonomous areas; whereas the 1978 constitution had only three articles outlining such forms, the new constitution has eleven. These articles introduce new responsibilities and obligations. As before, the number of national minority representatives is to be an "appropriate" number. However, article 113 states that either the chairman or the vice-chairman—or both—must be a citizen of the nationality or nationalities exercising autonomy. In fact, autonomous nationalities had usually been so represented, but they were now guaranteed one of the highest regional government posts by law for the first time.[7] Further, article 114 calls for the administrative head of an autonomous unit of government at the regional, prefectural, or county level to be a citizen of the nationality exercising autonomy in that area.

Other new provisions extended autonomous governments' authority over their own local affairs. Article 117 calls for revenues accruing to minority areas to be managed and used within the autonomous unit itself. Article 118 states that an autonomous area may independently arrange and administer local economic development. Article 119 specifically calls for the independent administration and development of such key areas as education and culture.[8] These three articles constitute a major departure from earlier constitutions with regard to the financial and cultural autonomy of minority areas, and they clearly demonstrate that reform has emphasized greater local and regional control over provincial-level affairs.

Policy has thus evolved from the CCP's earliest flirtations with self-determination in the 1930s to party- and state-guided autonomy and, most recently, to an autonomy that, on paper at least, approaches that promised minorities in the 1950s. It is important to remember, however, that power in China is vested in the CCP and the PLA; these remain largely the province of Han Chinese, despite efforts at minority recruitment. The primary role played by these two powerful institutions in minority areas has meant that Chinese have ultimately controlled the dimensions and pace of change.

The CCP's Role in National Minority Regions

The Chinese Communist Party presented itself not only as the victor in the struggle against imperialism and its lackeys, but also as the champion of minorities who had been equally oppressed by the rule of the Guomindang. In the new China, the CCP would provide leadership and social education for the minorities, guiding them toward a new socialist future.

In CCP discussions of minority nationalities, it is clear that the ultimate resolution of the national question lies in the eventual assimilation of all peoples into one great Chinese people. This is presented as a long-range goal, however, and party literature is clear in emphasizing that this will occur only after a very long period of time. In 1962, for example, national minorities' "special characteristics and national differences" were expected to exist throughout the evolutionary period of national minority societies—and "for a long historical period after the communist society has been reached."[9] An attempt was also made in the first two decades of CCP rule to distinguish CCP goals from those of the GMD. In 1958, the government addressed the issue of assimilationist policies, stressing once more the long-term nature of CCP policies and stating its strong opposition to the assimilationist stance of the Guomindang.[10]

While these statements attempted to distance the CCP's policy from that of the GMD, there are nonetheless some interesting similarities in the language and political slogans used to express the official party lines of both the GMD and the CCP. Both refer to minorities as *xiong di* (brothers). Han are often described as the elder brother, a relationship that implies responsibilities for the elder as well as the need for deference on the part of the younger—who owes lifelong respect and obedience to his elder brother. Referring to minorities as *didi* (younger brother) is thus far more paternalistic than it is fraternal, and has been a cause of resentment, especially among Muslim groups.

The inequality between the Han and minorities is reinforced in other ways. Like the GMD before them, the CCP consistently refers to the minority areas as *luohou* (backward), a term applied both to minority economic development and to minority culture. The lack of writing systems among some smaller minority groups and the "failure" to develop urban centers among others are two examples used to illustrate this backwardness. These provide a rationale for a greater Han Chinese presence in minority areas: The Han can help raise the cultural level of the people, while at the same time contributing to these areas' economic development. Like the GMD, the CCP uses the slogan *minzu tuanjie* (nationalities' unity) and consistently refers to the need for unity among all nationalities—Han and minority nationalities alike. These terms have marked Chinese rhetoric on minority issues since the 1950s.

Finally, in comparing the two parties' approaches to minority issues, both have publicly avowed their determination to guarantee personal freedoms to all China's minorities. Both parties have provided written guarantees of legal equality, of religious and cultural freedom, and of a certain degree of self-government for minority areas. The desirability of national minorities' direct participation in government and party organizations (and to a far less extent in the military) has been acknowledged by both, although the CCP's efforts in this area have been far more successful.

From 1949 onward, CCP policy has focused on the short-term goal of establishing the autonomy system as a basis for minority participation in government and political affairs—beginning the process of integration of minority areas into the Chinese economic and political system. But, in fact, implementation of even short-term measures has been inconsistent, often at variance with the official policy statements outlined above. The political upheavals of the 1950s and 1960s had a huge impact in minority areas and engendered further distrust of Chinese promises and guarantees of rights and freedoms. From the standpoint of many minorities, life under the CCP has meant continued uncertainty, as paper promises have been repeatedly set aside in the name of national political movements and as agendas for change have been prepared without reference to minority views.

PRC Nationalities Policy Implementation in Xinjiang, 1949–1996

The Early Years: 1949–1957

From 1949 to 1955, the administration of Xinjiang was in the hands of the region's new top military leaders, all Han Chinese. While the role of the military was also important elsewhere in China, the military in the northwest held greater power and held it far longer than in other areas. In theory, the military was there to establish order and to represent the authority of the new government in Beijing. It was to take control at every level, from the provincial government in Urumqi to the local, village level, where military-controlled committees were to work with local leaders to explain the nature of the revolution and the new government that would start all Chinese citizens down the socialist road. Liu Shaoqi, who was to become China's president from 1959 to 1966, described the process this way:

> The military control of the People's Liberation Army is the initial form of the dictatorship of the people's democracy, which suppresses the reactionaries by force and at the same time everywhere protects the people, inspires them, and helps them to set up Conferences of People's

Representatives, organs of the people's power at all levels, which, as conditions become ripe, are gradually given full power.[11]

As noted previously, Chinese descriptions of the process by which the PLA took power in minority areas invariably stress that it was, in general, a peaceful transfer of authority. Such is the usual characterization for that process in Xinjiang; references to the "peaceful liberation of Xinjiang" are a primary theme in Chinese accounts of this period.

These accounts note the important contribution to a peaceful transfer made by Burhan Shahidi, the GMD-appointed chairman of the provincial government, and by General Tao Zhiyue, the GMD's garrison commander for Xinjiang. These two leaders vacillated over what course of action to follow in the spring and summer of 1949. By August, they were conferring urgently with colleagues throughout the region before making their decision. On September 25, Tao sent a brief telegram to Chairman Mao, declaring his change of allegiance; the next day, Burhan followed suit. The approximately 100,000 GMD troops in the region were told to remain at their posts and await the arrival of the PLA. As the GMD troops controlled seven of the region's ten districts, the surrender of these men probably did ensure a transfer of power that was relatively peaceful. Certainly the combination of the GMD and the newly arrived, battle-hardened troops from China proper constituted an overwhelming military presence that would have made armed resistance extremely difficult in the oases. More passive resistance, in the form of noncompliance, obstruction, and so on, as well as covert acts of sabotage and assassination are probable, but sources thus far do not allow more than speculation about the incidence of these activities. Given that such resistance was commonplace against the GMD military, it would likely have continued after 1949 against the PLA.

Details on the first years of PLA rule in Xinjiang remain unavailable, but a reading of both Chinese and Western sources confirms that there was continued armed resistance, much of it in Kazak areas. In a series of what the new government referred to as "bandit-suppression campaigns," the PLA first isolated and then literally hunted down the small and poorly armed groups that had chosen to resist. Some may have had American encouragement—as GMD and CCP sources both suggest—but clearly they did not receive American military support.[12] Groups such as the one led by Osman Batur suffered more than they might have otherwise because of the suspicion that they had sought and/or received American support. In these tense, early years after the defeat of America's ally, Chiang Kaishek, and the beginning of the Korean War, the United States was considered a very real military threat to the new Chinese government. Any person or group associated with the United States provided evidence for a continued American influence on "counter-revolutionaries." The public execution of Osman and other leaders in 1951 was one means by which the reality of this threat could be given concrete form.

If a possible American-backed resistance provided one reason for a strong military presence in Xinjiang, the threat of USSR involvement provided another. Despite the fact that China and the USSR were allies, the CCP was keenly aware of past Russian influence in the region. "Isolated" Xinjiang was clearly not immune to the interests of the Great Powers, and the extreme force that was used there in the early years of the PRC is a reflection of this fact. Accusing resistance leaders of being the lackeys of foreign powers offered further justification for an especially heavy Chinese military presence.

Suggestions of foreign powers at work to counter the Chinese revolution also served to draw attention away from another, far more troubling problem—the East Turkestan Republic. As PLA troops entered the region from the east, the East Turkestani government in the Ili Valley remained in control of the three far northwestern districts of Xinjiang, the same districts that contained the majority of the region's Kazaks. More to the point, the republic also had an army of some 30,000 Uyghurs, Kazaks, ethnic Russians, and other minorities, all relatively well armed with Russian-made weapons and captured GMD guns.[13]

The presence of this armed force required a cautious approach during the first few months of PLA presence in Xinjiang. Recent Chinese sources declare that this army was peacefully incorporated into the PLA as the Fifth Army in the winter of 1949–1950. Western sources suggest that an agreement with the USSR facilitated the merger, but documentation is lacking. Regardless of how the union of the two forces was arranged, the Turkic Muslims of the East Turkestani military were, officially at least, incorporated into the PLA that first winter. The military now dealt quickly with any lingering threat; in 1950–1951, individual members of the new Fifth Army were transferred to posts throughout the region, while others were sent to eastern

China for further political and military training. At the same time, whole units of the Fifth Army were transferred out of the Ili area; several were assigned duties as part of the bandit-suppression campaigns of 1952–1953, particularly against Osman Batur.[14]

Several reports criticized the *minzujun* (nationalities army) soldiers of the Fifth Army as not adequately revolutionary and in need of stricter discipline. Breaking up the original units was one way of dealing with this, but these efforts must not have been deemed adequate, for in 1954 the Fifth Army was abruptly disbanded. By then the PLA was in control of all the major towns and villages, and controlled all transport and communication arteries. Although some more remote areas, such as the Tarbagatay and Altay Mountains, remained on the periphery of Chinese control, access to and from these regions was now in PLA hands. While the special, local knowledge of the minzujun units had been no doubt useful in the early years, continued difficulty in dealing with this inadequately revolutionary unit probably contributed to the Chinese decision to disband the Fifth Army.

While the military's role in gaining control of the region was paramount, the party was simultaneously laying the foundations for a new government at the regional and local levels. In an effort to overcome distrust of Han Chinese intentions, the CCP and the PLA sought cooperation of local leaders. A "united front" policy included the retention of GMD-appointed officials. Burhan, the last governor under the GMD, continued in his post. In recognition of the importance of the Ili region, his deputy governor was Saifudin Azizi (Seypidin), who had been a member of the coalition government of 1946–1947. The GMD-appointed commander Tao also remained in Xinjiang, now serving as second in command of the region's military forces.

At the highest government levels, however, there was no proportionate national minority representation, leaving the promises of the Common Program unfulfilled. In Xinjiang, each national minority was given at least one representative on the government council; Uyghurs, who constituted 75 percent of the population, held only 29 percent of council seats. When the council was subsequently enlarged to seventy-one members, Uyghurs held twenty-four seats, or 34 percent. Han Chinese, who were then about 6 percent of the region's population, held fifteen seats, or 21 percent. The remaining positions were held by representatives of the remaining nationalities.

By 1953, the process of identifying China's minorities and accord-

Table 4.1

Autonomous Prefectures (A.P.) and Autonomous Counties (A.C.) in Xinjiang in the mid-1950s

Autonomous Unit	Number of Nationalities	Largest Nationality
Barkol-Kazak (A.C.)	8	Kazak, 31%
Bayangol-Mongol (A.P.)	12	Mongol, 35%
Bortala-Mongol (A.P.)	13	Mongol, 25%
Changji-Hui (A.P.)	11	Hui, 37%
Hobosar-Mongol (A.C.)	7	Mongol, 58%
Ili-Kazak (A.P.)	12	Kazak, 53%
Kizilsu-Kirghiz (A.P.)	11	Kirghiz, 36%
Mori-Kazak (A.C.)	9	Kazak, 33%
Qapqal-Xibo (A.C.)	6	Xibo, 28%
Tashkorgan-Tajik (A.C.)	6	Tajik, 38%
Yanqi-Hui (Karashar) (A.C.)	8	Hui, 33%

ing them official national minority status had led to the recognition of thirteen nationalities in Xinjiang.[15] Seven of these—the Mongols, Kirghiz, Hui, Kazaks, Tajiks, Xibo, and Uyghurs—had been given some form of autonomous government by 1954. In recognition of the predominance of the Uyghurs, the region was ultimately renamed the Xinjiang-Uyghur Autonomous Region in 1955. As table 4.1 indicates, all of the lower-level autonomous units have between six and thirteen different nationalities, and only in two does a single group constitute a majority. The system precludes any particular group from claiming dominance. This arrangement can be seen as recognition of the multi-ethnic composition of much of the region, but in some instances it appears that the government created counties and prefectures that would be sure to include a number of different nationalities. The Ili-Kazak Autonomous Prefecture, for instance, was further subdivided into autonomous counties in a way that is quite unlike any other area of Xinjiang. As this was the territory that had seceded from China in 1945 and that had retained its independence until 1949, the special adminis-trative structure appears directly related to this area's separatist history.

Once the lower levels of government were organized, the autono-mous regional government itself was established on October 1, 1955. The first chairman was Saifudin Azizi, the Uyghur from the Ili area who had participated in the Three Districts Revolution of 1944. The new standing committee of the regional people's congress had forty-four members, thirty-three of whom were representatives of the region's nationalities; but as with earlier governmental bodies, the Uyghurs, who were still clearly the dominant majority in the region, remained a minority in the government. Their nineteen seats gave them 46 percent of the total. Han Chinese held 19.5 percent, and other nationalities divided the remained 34 percent. Although in fact the power of these bodies was limited and subject to the policies formulated in Beijing by the CCP, central government concern for the appearance of following its own guidelines for autonomous areas took second place to greater concerns of national security and, it must be assumed, distrust even of the modest CCP minority cohort that was emerging in Xinjiang in the 1950s.

As the CCP held ultimate authority everywhere in China, it was important from the outset for the party to cultivate members of all national minorities to serve in the party apparatus at all levels. But the highest party positions at all levels invariably belonged to Han Chinese. Han dominance has persisted especially in border regions like Xinjiang, where both international and domestic groups have been accused of stirring up animosity toward the party.[16] In Xinjiang the top CCP post was held by Wang Enmao. He had come to Xinjiang initially with Wang Zhen, commander of the First Army Corps in Xinjiang from 1949 to 1952. Under Wang Zhen, Wang Enmao was based in Kashgar; his role there is officially considered to have been an important one, yet Chinese sources provide very little information on what he actually did. On the other hand, anecdotal information from Uyghurs and other minorities in Xinjiang at the time uniformly depict him in a strongly negative light, which is not surprising since the arrival of yet another Chinese military force cannot have been very welcome in Kashgar, regardless of how good the intentions of that force ostensibly were.[17] In 1952, the CCP promoted Wang Zhen, moving him from Xinjiang to Beijing. Wang Enmao then moved from Kashgar to Urumqi, where he became the highest party official in the region. His success in Xinjiang contributed to his being appointed a full member of the CCP's central committee in 1956.

Official reports on PLA and CCP work in the Xinjiang region during these early years are almost all very positive, reflecting more the revolutionary rhetoric required by the times than the actual situation in the region. By 1955, however, even official reports gave some indication of dissatisfaction among the local Muslim population; and by the time of the Hundred Flowers campaign in the spring of 1957, this dissatisfaction with the role of the party was being expressed publicly. In May of that year, criticism of the party unleashed by Chairman Mao's call for open discussion of the party's progress, included sharp criticism of the overwhelming presence of Han cadres. For example, a minority cadre named Hussein was quoted as saying, "The problem in existence is that at present there are not enough nationalities cadres but too many Han cadres. I wanted to say something in this connection but because of my fear of the charge of local nationalism, I did not raise the question."[18] Another minority cadre claimed that "in actual work there is the phenomenon for the Han nationality cadres to accept the tasks assigned to them without implementing them."[19]

In the autumn of 1957, Deng Xiaoping announced that minority regions of China would also participate in the national "rectification" campaign already well launched elsewhere in China. In Xinjiang, the dual focus of this campaign was on counterrevolutionaries and on "local nationalism"—the twin evils against which the local population needed to be mobilized. Han chauvinism, which was not to be tolerated according to earlier party directives, was not emphasized—despite clear indications in the minority comments released during the Hundred Flowers that there were still considerable problems in this area. In October 1957, a judicial work conference was convened, the goal of which was to organize a winter campaign against all bad elements in the region. These included not only local nationalists, but also criminal elements who were said to be active in several areas, most notably in Yining, the capital of the Ili-Kazak Autonomous Prefecture. A November 1957 report condemned a counterrevolutionary organization in Xinjiang called the China Peasant Party, which was said to operate among the men in the labor reform camps and was reportedly planning a general mass uprising in the region.[20] "China peasant" is a phrase that suggests such a party would be largely Han, rather than local and Muslim. It is certainly possible that such a group had been organized among the demobilized GMD troops who were assigned work not unlike that done by the men in labor reform camps; if so, the group could certainly have been counterrevolutionary. But once again, there is little corroboration thus far about the nature of this group or its purported activities.

Much more troubling to the authorities was increased agitation for greater autonomy by local minority groups. A demand had been made, for instance, that there be separate communist parties for each national-ity, a request clearly unacceptable to the CCP, as were also demands that Han cadre and Han settlers leave Xinjiang. Finally, and certainly most threatening to the government, were calls for the formation of a new and independent East Turkestan.[21] The identity of those request-ing these radical changes remains unclear. Although the CCP identi-fied such individuals by an array of epithets ranging from "bad elements" to "national splittists," details on the number of individuals involved or on what groups provided leadership were not given in press reports, which invariably conveyed an image of small and pow-erless groups that nonetheless threatened national security and that, therefore, required total eradication. In some instances, the Chinese authorities also blamed unidentified, outside agitators, following the GMD's earlier policy that blamed all internal difficulties in Xinjiang on the USSR.

A more likely source of opposition was the largely urban, educated elite. An article published in April 1958 intended to rebut Xinjiang's local nationalists noted that some of the region's agitators were basing their renewed claim for self-determination on Marxism. These critics were suggesting that the Soviet system could serve as a model for the CCP: "The nationalists argue that the establishment of an Uighuristan [sic] or an Uighur Republic does not necessarily mean its separation from China, but that it may form a part of the Chinese union. They think that . . . since the Soviet Union adopts such a system it should be followed in China."[22] Such arguments appear to be those of a rela-tively educated group, aware of the differences in Chinese and Soviet communism and having a fair knowledge of the constitutions of the two states. By 1958, however, the political climate in China had shifted again, and local demands were once more subsumed in a rapid push to communization.

The Great Leap Forward and Its Aftermath

While debate on the issue of nationalism in Xinjiang continued, the CCP began its drive to establish communes throughout China as part of Mao's Great Leap Forward, which began in 1958. The central gov-ernment demanded that Xinjiang conform fully to this and other na-tional-level policies. The policy of recognizing minority areas' special characteristics, which had allowed for a slower pace of change in such regions, was abandoned. To strengthen regional compliance, the numbers of young Han Chinese being sent out to border areas increased. A steady stream of these newest settlers began entering Xinjiang.[23]

The new settlers, coupled with the requirement that Xinjiang participate fully in the party's attempt to jumpstart the Chinese economy, brought increased tensions. As is true of other particularly sensitive periods of Xinjiang's modern history, there are few details on the events of the bitter years of 1959–1962. Refugees would later tell of long bread lines and food shortages; although the area did not evidently see the level of famine that struck other parts of China, even the usually productive Ili Valley saw extreme shortages. Political repression also increased during these years, leading many local Muslims to emigrate across the border into the USSR.

As emigration escalated, the authorities abruptly decided to close the border. In 1962 a mass exodus of thousands of Kazaks and Uyghurs triggered the Yi-Ta incident in the city of Yining, where in late May 1962 Chinese troops fired into a crowd of demonstrators who were demanding the right to leave China. An unknown number of people were killed and the border was closed. (See chapter 5 for further discussion of this incident.)

The official PRC press made no mention of the incident at the time. Estimates of people fleeing CCP rule as a result of deprivations in the Ili-Kazak area range from 60,000 to over 100,000. Rather than interpreting this as a local response to unsuccessful policies of the Great Leap, the government ultimately linked the exodus of 1962 to outside interference. Unwilling to take responsibility for this rapid depopulation of several border counties in a matter of a few months, the events of 1962 were instead added to the list of grievances against the Soviet Union.[24]

As elsewhere in China, after 1962 there was a return to more moderate policies. In Xinjiang, minority policy once again tolerated aspects of Muslim culture. Muslim religious festivals, the celebration of which had been reported in the press every year prior to the beginning of the Great Leap in 1958, were once again well publicized. For instance, in 1964, a three-day religious holiday was announced, and heavy attendance at local mosques was reported in the local press.[25]

In the period of 1962–1965, Xinjiang's party leader Wang Enmao was strengthening his own position. He was already the first secretary of the local party; in February 1964 he became secretary of the CCP's Northwest China Bureau. A year later he was named as a member of the National Defense Council, partly in recognition of his region's "front-line" position on the sensitive Soviet border. In March 1966, his status was further enhanced with an appointment as first secretary of the PCC.

By 1965, Saifudin had been chairman of the region for more than ten years.[26] During this decade Xinjiang had experienced great changes, especially in economic development. The region's total grain production, for instance, was reported as having risen from 2,035,273,000 catties in 1949[27] to 6,105,819,000 in 1965.[28] Cash income reportedly rose three times over the preliberation level,[29] while retail prices for manufactured goods dropped four times between 1956 and 1964.[30] Land-reclamation and water-conservancy projects had been carried out by the government, using mostly Han Chinese labor, and huge state farms had been built, primarily in northern Xinjiang, on lands that included former pasturage but also marginal lands laboriously reclaimed by the paramilitary force of the PCC. Industry, too, had been launched in the region: From an estimated total industrial production of 81 million yuan in 1949, output increased to 636 million yuan by 1965.[31]

Saifudin described these changes as "earth shaking"; certainly the region had changed dramatically in the decade since it had become the Xinjiang-Uyghur Autonomous Region. But not all these changes were viewed as positive by the local population, and tensions between nationalities continued on the eve of the Cultural Revolution. Thus while Saifudin praised the economic changes that had occurred, he also warned his fellow Uyghurs and other minorities of the dangers of "local nationalism." He condemned those who advocated the reestablishment of the Communist Party in Xinjiang along national lines. He called for increased recruitment of national minority cadres as one means of safeguarding Xinjiang, declaring that this would protect the region from Soviet efforts "to split Xinjiang from the great Fatherland."[32]

Saifudin's speech strongly suggested that despite economic advances—and despite efforts at recruiting a minority cadre to serve in the CCP—dissatisfaction with their new government and the CCP remained a problem among the Xinjiang region's minorities in 1965.

Xinjiang and the Cultural Revolution, 1966–1976

Officially, the Cultural Revolution began in Xinjiang on August 3, 1966, with a broadcast by Zhou Enlai over Radio Urumqi, asking the people of Xinjiang for their support in the Great Proletarian Cultural Revolution. A month later, Urumqi welcomed 400 newly arrived Han Chinese Red Guards. The following day, a serious incident occurred involving local Muslims and these young "revolutionaries."[33] Wang Enmao was suspected of orchestrating the incident in order to discredit the Red Guard movement and, possibly, to keep the movement out of the region altogether. If such was the case, he was not immediately successful, for Red Guard units continued to arrive.

As these numbers grew, factions developed, as they did elsewhere in China. The main division was between supporters and opponents of Wang, who held the loyalties of many leading Han Chinese officials in the region. The pro-Wang groups included the Xinjiang Red Revolutionary Rebel First Headquarters and the PCC's August First Field Army Swearing to Defend the Thought of Mao Zedong to the Death.[34]

Initially, Wang had the upper hand. Angered by the introduction of the Cultural Revolution into Xinjiang—a region that was already tense without the added element of the radical Red Guard units—Wang traveled to Beijing in December 1966. His efforts there were successful, for on January 26, 1967, the military commission of the Central Committee decided that areas on "China's first line of defense" should postpone the Cultural Revolution.[35] A month later, Zhou Enlai himself called for an end to the Cultural Revolution in Xinjiang. By March, the Chinese press praised Wang Enmao as a true follower of Mao; it appeared that he had successfully halted the Cultural Revolution in his region.

But the forces unleashed in 1966 were not so easily deflected. In the summer of 1967, there were violent and bloody clashes in Xinjiang. Red Guard bulletins claimed that truckloads of bodies were hauled away after clashes between the pro-Wang August First Field Army and anti-Wang Red Guard units from outside the region.[36]

Tensions continued in the winter of 1967–1968. Early in 1968, Saifudin, the regional chairman, became the object of Red Guard attacks. After the chairman's house was ransacked, Zhou Enlai again intervened directly, reprimanding members of the Red Second Headquarters reportedly responsible for the incident.[37] Undaunted, the Red Guards then turned on other Muslim targets, focusing on the Uyghur vice-chairman, Iminov, and Burhan Shahidi, the Tatar ex-governor of the region. Both men were repeatedly attacked in the local press and were subsequently stripped of their posts. Like other high officials who ran afoul of the Red Guards, both men disappeared from public view.

While leaders of provinces and regions all over China were being demoted or were disappearing altogether, both Wang Enmao and Saifudin seemed inviolate. In 1968, when the region announced the formation of the Xinjiang Revolutionary Committee, a new ruling body vested with all previous governmental power, both Wang and Saifudin were listed as members, and both remained on government rosters as "responsible persons." Although a new military commander was assigned to Xinjiang, Long Shujin, the "old guard" of Wang and Saifudin retained their positions.

The continued presence of Saifudin as a regional government and party official did not prevent attacks on religion, however. Zealous Red Guards saw Islam as a holdover from feudal society and condemned it as one of the "four olds." Copies of the Koran were reportedly burned; mosques and Muslim cemeteries were desecrated.[38] The public observance of Muslim holidays and festivals such as Kurban-bairam (the feast of Ibrahim) and Ramadan were abolished. Destruction of mosques was widespread, and in many towns and villages religious leaders were detained. The pilgrimages to Mecca that had begun on a small scale in the 1950s and early 1960s also ended; they were not resumed until 1980.[39] The Xinjiang branch of China's Islamic Association disappeared, resuming public activities only in the early 1980s.

In the summer of 1969, international developments finally ended the Cultural Revolution in Xinjiang. In December 1968 there had been violent clashes with the USSR military near the city of Tacheng on the northwest border of Xinjiang. In May and June 1969, once the worst of the winter weather subsided, clashes marked by heavy artillery fire resumed in the same area.[40] This international threat to China's national security took precedence over domestic politics, and the Cultural Revolution was declared over.

The worst violence and excesses of the Cultural Revolution diminished in 1969–1970, but concern over the role of religious leaders in Xinjiang society remained, as did concern over the possibility of the USSR's exploiting internal problems in the region to its advantage.

The official rhetoric conveying this concern referred repeatedly to "national splittists" and "Soviet revisionists." In 1975, the Xinjiang press was still referring to "a handful of national splittist elements and counterrevolutionaries under the cloak of religion who throw themselves into the arms of Soviet revisionists."[41]

Although the movement officially ended in 1969, reorganization of the region's government and party apparatus took time to complete. In 1973, Long Shujin, the military leader transferred to the area in 1968, was removed from his post as head of the Xinjiang Revolutionary Committee and replaced by Saifudin. The following year, Saifudin was named first secretary of the party and first political commissar of the PLA in Xinjiang, and he remained chairman of the Xinjiang Revolutionary Committee. His political stature was further enhanced when he was made an alternate to the politburo of the Central Committee and a vice-chairman of the standing committee of the National People's Congress. Wang Enmao also survived the political storm, once more being named first secretary of the party in Xinjiang in 1981.

Mao's death in 1976 marked the end of a decade-long period of political intolerance of minorities' differing cultural and religious practices. After 1976, party and media rhetoric once more referred to the special characteristics of China's minority nationalities, and a new attempt to win the loyalties of the minorities began.

Xinjiang in the Reform Era, 1978–1996

In Xinjiang, one measure of the policy shift after 1976 was the increasing number of minorities appearing in government posts. For example, of eleven vice-chairmen serving in the regional government under Saifudin in 1973, only two were minorities: Ismayil Aymat, Uyghur, and Zuya, a Kazak. But in 1978, when the regional people's congress convened under Han Chinese chairman Wang Feng, five of the thirteen vice-chairmen were national minorities.[42]

In the 1980s, efforts continued to promote national minority cadre to higher government posts. The 1979 and 1983 regional people's congresses were both convened by a Uyghur chairman, Tomor Dawamut. Fully half of the vice-chairmen were national minorities. The provincial government officials elected by these two assemblies reflected a similar proportion of Han to minority nationalities: The 1979 regional government, for example, was led by a Uyghur, Ismayil Aymat, and six of his twelve vice-chairmen were minorities; Ismayil's 1983 government included only six vice-chairmen, but once again the fifty-fifty ratio was followed, with three Han and three minorities. At lower levels of government, all the chairmen of the standing committees and many of the leadership posts were held by national minorities, except in the far northwestern part of Xinjiang.[43]

The 1980s also saw renewed concern over the drop in numbers of minority cadre and CCP members. Prior to the Cultural Revolution, the number of such cadre personnel had grown from 12,841 in 1950 to 106,000 in 1965.[44] However, after the Cultural Revolution, the number had fallen below 80,000.[45] By 1979, national minorities accounted for only 29 percent of the region's total cadre. Efforts began to increase these numbers, and by 1983 there were reportedly 181,860 national minority cadres, an increase of 75,000 from 1965. In part, the rapid rejuvenation evidenced by these numbers was a result of the reinstatement of cadres expelled unjustly during the Cultural Revolution.[46] By 1990, the CCP claimed a total of 225,000 minority cadre, or 46 percent of the region's total. The government also asserted that 65 percent of the members on the standing committee of the regional people's congress were minorities, as were 64 percent of the regional government staff.[47]

The above indicators are important evidence of the trend in minority affairs since 1980. For most of the region's Muslims, however, the return to an earlier era of respect for religious and cultural practices was of greater import. Not only were mosques once again opened for worship, but, in some instances, the government also provided funds for the repair and reconstruction of structures damaged by the Red Guards in the 1960s. Religious holidays were once more observed, and local Han Chinese leaders extended appropriate good wishes to the Muslim population on these occasions. Muslim workers again enjoyed days off work for the public observance of Kurban-bairam and Ramadan. Goods specifically for Muslims—and other national minorities—reappeared in department stores.

In 1980, the government's efforts to impose a romanized form of Uyghur and Kazak script were abandoned; a modified Arabic script returned to the schools and popular use. Publishing shifted to the Arabic script in the early 1980s, and by the end of the decade books in the romanized forms of Uyghur and Kazak disappeared from bookstores.

These restored freedoms were accompanied by the dismantling of the old commune system throughout the region and by the advent of a more open economy. The process of ending the commune system took longer in Xinjiang, however, than in China proper. As late as 1985, government reports stated that the region had "basically completed" the work of separating government administration from commune management, a description that implied only a partial change to the new economic system.[48] "Free" markets emerged in towns throughout the region in the early 1980s; by the middle of the decade, open-air stalls in cities and larger towns sold a wide variety of goods, ranging from imported blue jeans and western-style clothes from Taiwan to more traditional Khotan carpets and Kashgar knives. Homegrown produce, spices, and meats appeared in abundance at competitive prices.

Accompanying these changes in the region's economic organization was a new policy called "opening up" to the outside. Trade with neighboring regions and states expanded, and improvements to the region's transport system reflected the government's interest in fostering trade. Connections to some of the major cities of China proper already existed via the railroad, which, however, ended at the regional capital, Urumqi. In 1991, work to extend the railroad to the Kazakstani border in the west was completed, and service began in 1992, adding a new transport artery and encouraging a lively border trade (see discussion in chapter 7). The Kunjerab Highway, linking southern Xinjiang and Pakistan, had been completed earlier, allowing a small boom in trade each summer season, despite recurring problems with landslides and inclement weather that virtually closed the highway during the long winter months.

Improvements in transportation not only aided in economic expansion, but also boosted tourism. By 1984, only a few years after the region was opened to individual travel, the city of Urumqi welcomed some 13,000 tourists.[49] In addition to the often overcrowded trains, tourists could take one of several flights a week that linked Beijing and Urumqi. With the decentralization of Civil Aviation Authority of China (CAAC), China's national air carrier, in the late 1980s, a new entity, Xinjiang Airlines, was established, providing a daily flight to and from Beijing and improving air connections between Urumqi and other cities in Xinjiang. By 1996, the Urumqi airport also boasted international flights, including destinations such as Moscow, Islamabad, Tashkent, and Almaty.

At the end of the twentieth century, no longer isolated from either China proper or neighboring states—which, after 1991, included Muslim countries of the former USSR—Xinjiang was in a position to reap the varied benefits of China's expanding economy. However, the role of the Kazaks and other Muslims in Xinjiang's new, increasingly Han-dominated society remains problematic. While some Kazaks are embracing change, as will be seen in subsequent chapters, the degree of Kazak participation in the new Xinjiang has been shaped by their past experiences under the PRC and by their reluctance to support and contribute to a region that will soon be only half Muslim.

In order to better understand Kazak circumstances in the 1990s, we will first survey the impact of the PRC's policies since 1949 on the Kazaks as a people. This discussion also provides background for the more detailed examination of Kazak areas in Xinjiang, which follows in chapter 5.

Xinjiang's Kazak Areas: An Overview of 1949–1996

The account of liberation in the pastoral areas of Xinjiang remains incomplete. A limited number of Chinese sources provide sketchy information on some of the events of the early years in Kazak areas, while refugee reports from the period offer further glimpses of the changeover in government. Reports by the last foreign officials in the area in 1949–1951 augment our knowledge; however, until extensive oral histories can be compiled and still-closed archives opened, only a partial account of the Kazaks during the early years of Chinese communist rule can be provided here.

Although the standard Chinese characterization is that Xinjiang experienced "peaceful liberation" in 1949, official Chinese sources and refugee accounts clearly indicate armed resistance in pastoral areas. The most determined resistance was presented by groups of Kazaks opposed to communist rule, as discussed in chapter 3; but the Kazaks were not united in their response to the PRC, and met it in many ways, ranging from cooperation to violent opposition.

Armed resistance was the choice of some. Osman, Janimhan, and other Kazak leaders reportedly led over 4,000 men, and these comprised the core of military opposition in the years 1949–1951.[50] In response, the PLA inaugurated a prolonged military action known as the "movement to suppress counter-revolutionaries," which lasted from 1950 to 1952; at the same time, the official CCP policy of "political struggle, military suppression" was carried out in the pastoral regions.[51] As a result of the campaigns associated with this policy, the PLA captured and executed Kazak and other minority leaders. According to the new government, these leaders' crimes ranged from murder and destruction of property to "estrangement of nationalities" in Xinjiang. In addition to the infamous Osman Batur, who was captured and executed in 1951, Kazak leaders Ali Beg Hakim and Janimhan were also identified as part of a United States-Guomindang special task force that was fomenting antirevolutionary disturbances, especially in the pastoral areas and near Changji, a town not far from the capital of Urumqi.[52] Official PRC histories stress that these and other renegade groups were defeated by 1952. If so, it took the combined force of hardened PLA troops and recruits from the army of the former East Turkestan Republic—possibly augmented by men from the thousands of GMD troops still in Xinjiang—to track down and defeat a relatively small number of rebels. The final official tally was 576 "bandit" leaders killed, 3,351 captured, and 4,000 surrendered. In addition, some 100,000 animals were recovered.[53]

Such open defiance was only one of several options chosen by Kazaks and other "pastoralists."[54] Some Kazaks who, like Osman, had been sympathetic to the GMD chose to leave the region altogether. Between 1949 and 1952, small groups of Kazak families made the difficult journey across mountain ranges into neighboring Pakistan, while a hardy few fled to Afghanistan.

Another option for pro-GMD Kazaks was to follow the example of a few Uyghur leaders in Urumqi and publicly accept the new government and its representatives. Groups that had previously opposed the PLA were pardoned upon their "surrender" if they could substantiate "meritorious service" to their own people. If they were accused of criminal activity, they could still be pardoned if they were willing to offer compensation for their crimes. Some also evidently were able to convince the PLA that they had been forced to participate in counterrevolutionary activities and should, therefore, be pardoned.[55] Although the PLA and the newly arrived Chinese officials must have been suspicious of some of these claims and changes in allegiance, it was initially to their advantage to accept some Kazak leaders, as part of the larger process of establishing CCP legitimacy in the region. Thus, for instance, the CCP welcomed former GMD district officer Hadewan, the wife of Kazak leader Alin Wang, into the government as a representative of the Kazaks despite her past party affiliation.

Finally, and perhaps more commonly, there was simple passive resistance, with some Kazak families retreating back into the most remote mountains. Even when CCP cadre were able to find them, persuading them to support "new China" was not an easy task. An anecdote often recounted about this period was that when two Chinese cadre reached a Kazak camp in the early 1950s, they called all the people together in order to explain the new government policies. The assembled group listened politely and, after providing a feast for the visitors in accordance with traditional Kazak hospitality, they offered the two men a place to sleep for the night. Satisfied with their day's work, the two cadre slept well; but when they awoke they discovered that the whole group of Kazaks had decamped in the night.[56]

As indicated earlier, it does not appear that the CCP was initially guided by specific policy in the early years of its dealings with the Kazaks. After all, the party's only experience with minorities from Xinjiang was the very limited connection they had established with some Uyghur leaders of the former East Turkestan Republic in 1947, a connection that was renewed only in August 1949. In 1950, the party had adopted the principle of "democratic consultation" for the pastoral areas. This meant that before proceeding with specific policies, cadre were to consult with Kazak leaders to determine local attitudes. Persuasion rather than force was to be used to introduce the new government to the Kazaks. By 1952, refinements to this general policy were needed. With direct experience now under its collective belt, the party formulated more specific guidelines for cadre in pastoral areas. These guidelines were encapsulated in the slogan of "three nos and two benefits." The three nos were *bu dou, bu fen,* and *buhuajieji*: no struggle, no redistribution, and no differentiation between classes. In other words, exempt from policies of struggle and class division pursued in Han Chinese peasant areas, the Kazak people would not have to undergo struggle meetings, nor would there be any immediate attempt to redistribute property or grazing rights. With little knowledge of "class structure" among the Kazaks and a paucity of Marxian wisdom to guide policy dealing with nomads, the party would not only ignore class divisions, but also, according to the "two benefits" principle, would provide benefits "to both herders and herd owners." In other words, only once pacification and military control of Kazak areas was accomplished would the work of education and persuasion begin.

Aid extended to the Kazaks in this early period focused on enhancing and increasing animal herds, the mainstay of Kazak life. The government began work on preventing diseases, killing wolves and rodents, cutting fodder for animals as winter feed, loaning money, and establishing co-ops that would buy the herders' products. Tax reforms were initiated. Reportedly, half of the herders were exempt from any tax, while the rest had their taxes lowered. According to a refugee from the Ili Valley area, during the first few years no one spoke of communism, only of democracy.[57]

Another potent means of persuasion was monetary. According to a Russian source, the CCP gave Xinjiang herders grants totaling over 14 billion yuan between 1949 and 1953.[58] If this amount is correct, it represents a huge investment for a country still undergoing reconstruction from the ravages of war. No details are available on how such funds might have been spent, but the amount suggests the possibility of payments to Kazak and other leaders, as well as support for military action and the purchase of animals from China's ally, the USSR.

Such policies bore fruit. Rather than killing their flocks and herds to avoid confiscation by the new government, as happened in the USSR during intensive collectivization, the number of animals in Xinjiang during the first four years of the PRC increased from 11.8 million to 15.4 million in 1953.[59]

While government activities in pastoral areas in the period 1949–1955 were largely pragmatic, an indication of longer term objectives appeared in 1953, after the suppression campaigns were officially over. In that year, the administrative committee for northwest China ordered that Xinjiang's Kazaks be given monetary aid to assist them in their transition away from nomadism and toward a settled life. Possibly under advice from the USSR, the CCP saw this transition as a necessary prerequisite for the development of socialism in Xinjiang. Thus, in an ironic imitation of the GMD's grants of money to the Kazak areas in 1946–1947, 12 billion yuan were allotted to the Kazaks of Xinjiang in 1953–1954. In the next two years, an additional 2.7 million yuan were allotted as loans to buy sheep. The increasing herds meant that by 1956, Xinjiang sheep supplied 60 percent of all China's wool.[60]

The large sums of money granted to "herders" between 1949 and 1954 not only may have been used to ensure Kazak cooperation with the new government; it also may have served to forestall any Soviet machinations among the Kazaks. But it is also likely that some of this money went to the PCC, a paramilitary organization that incorporated much of the surrendered GMD force into its many work units. By 1955, the PCC operated sixteen of its own livestock farms, most of them north of the Tian Shan. These former soldiers, new to animal husbandry, had to acquire stock as the basis for what became huge state-run enterprises by the end of the decade. Some of the funds mentioned above were thus possibly paid to Kazaks for their herds, providing a basis for the PCC's own livestock operations. Funds also may have gone to the new state-run stock farms—forty-two of which were established in addition to those of the PCC.[61] Extending financial aid was one means of persuading Kazaks to support—or, at least, not to oppose—the new government; the CCP also viewed the holding of elections as another means of establishing its legitimacy and authority. Local elections were held as early as March 1950 in some parts of Xinjiang, thereby establishing district and *xiang* (township) government units, as well as street committees in the towns and village of more rural areas. By 1951, the Xinjiang Province First All Nationalities People's Representative Congress was held in Urumqi, with 549 people from all minority nationalities attending.[62] On paper, the democratic principle was already at work.

However, official Chinese sources also state that while elections were held "almost everywhere" in the region by 1954, elections in some Kazak areas had to be delayed. A Soviet source on the period noted the following reason:

> This [lack of elections] is explained by the fact that here the necessary conditions had not been created and socialist transformation had hardly been carried out, because these districts are cattle-raising and semi-cattle-raising districts.[63]

Elections constituted an initial step in introducing the new socialist order to Kazak areas, but equally important were the moves toward collective ownership that began in 1952 with the formation of mutual-aid teams. In Kazak areas near the provincial capital, mutual-aid teams were formed more or less on schedule in 1952, but in the Ili-Kazak area progress was decidedly slow, with the first teams forming only in 1956.

As elsewhere in China and in Xinjiang's farming districts, the mutual-aid teams gave way to cooperatives, described as state-private cooperatives for herders. By 1958, in conformity with the national push to communes, the pastoral areas were also required to organize into communes, twenty-four of which were established in 1958. These incorporated 86 percent of the herders, according to PRC sources. In some areas, however, joint state-private enterprises continued to exist.[64]

By autumn of 1959, official reports from Xinjiang claimed that the process of transforming the "feudal nomadic system" to a socialist economy was "basically complete." Saifudin, the chairman of the regional government, explained the course of the process from its beginning stages to the formation of the communes in this way:

> With regard to the transformation of the herd-owner economy, we have adopted a policy of "buying out" the capital of the herd owners, in accordance with which the public-private jointly operated stock farms were formed, with the private herd owners retaining their shares in these farms and receiving dividends out of these shares. After the establishment of the people's communes, these shares of animals were converted into money at a certain price and a fixed interest was paid the private owners and the private owners were given suitable jobs in the farms. After a suitable period, all these public-private jointly operated stock farms will be gradually transformed into state-owned farms. With regard to the transformation of the individual economy of the herdsman, the same measures as taken in agricultural cooperativization were adopted. The animals owned by these herdsmen were pooled together in cooperatives and the profits were shared among the herdsmen according to the number of animals and amount of work they had contributed to the pool. Subsequently, their animals were bought by the communes at a certain price.[65]

As a result of this cautious procedure, Saifudin noted that the transition to the new economic form had been smooth and that losses were avoided and herd expansion encouraged.

However, figures for the total number of animals in Xinjiang in these early stages of socialist transformation only partially support Saifudin's assessment. Between 1949 and 1957, the total number of animals

Table 4.2

Total Livestock in Xinjiang 1943–1992

Year	Number of Livestock
1943	14,430,000
1949	12,000,000
1953	15,430,000
1954	17,100,000
1957	20,460,000
1959	22,230,000
1965	24,200,000
1974	27,900,000
1980	26,730,000
1983	30,240,000
1985	35,388,000
1992	34,940,000

Sources: The 1943 figure is from Lattimore, *Pivot of Asia,* 155. Figures for 1949 to 1985 are from *Xinjiang-Weiwuer zizhiqu gaikuang* (1985); *Mulei Hasake zizhixian gaikuang* (1984); and *Balikun Hasake zizhixian gaikuang* (1984). The 1992 figure is from *Xinjiang nianjian 1992* (Xinjiang yearbook 1992), 211.

in the region grew by about a million a year, a growth that, as discussed earlier, may have been heavily subsidized by central government payments. But for the years after the push toward communes, from 1958 to 1965, the total increase was only 2 million, or an average of some 250,000 a year (see table 4.2). Other causes can be suggested for this slowdown, from the economic crisis that marked the beginning of the Great Leap Forward in 1958 to underreporting—a not-unlikely phenomenon at a time when the government was requiring that all flocks and herds be merged as part of the new push toward socialism. Nonetheless, it is of interest to note that while Saifudin praised the economic transformation, the figures the government itself released allow a less optimistic assessment.

In the late 1950s and early 1960s, the official Chinese media attempted to present a rosy picture of the efforts to settle Kazaks in new villages, ending their nomad life. Reports described in detail how the happy villagers received the benefits of education and medical care once they settled. The former hardships suffered due to their nomadic existence had disappeared in the new lifestyle so earnestly advocated by the government. However, like Saifudin's remarks on the process of communization, these reports were also at variance with political developments between 1958 and 1965. In 1958, minority leaders of the recently established Ili-Kazak Autonomous Prefecture were purged. The highest Kazak official ousted was the chairman of the prefecture, Yahuda.

Other indicators of the shift in PRC policy toward minorities included a change in the legal marriage age: In January 1959 the government announced that the prefecture would now conform to the new, national law that stipulated legal marriage ages as twenty for men and eighteen for women. Previously, in keeping with the right of autonomous governments to pass laws in accord with local conditions, the ages in Xinjiang were lower—eighteen for men and sixteen for women—although marriages were often negotiated at even earlier ages in accordance with tradition. In addition to raising the marriage age, monogamy was to be enforced, as was the right of women to seek divorce. Officially, these changes were "spontaneously sought" by the masses.[66] However, as earlier marriage evidently continued despite the laws, and as monogamy was traditionally the rule among Kazaks, publicity for these "changes" apparently made little difference in Kazak areas.

During these years, economic conditions deteriorated, even in the usually fertile and productive Ili Valley. As will be recounted in chapter 5, shortages of staples like flour occurred, leading to long queues outside local shops and bakeries. The drive for conformity with national policies and the harshness with which this was pursued contributed to the 1962 exodus.

A major factor in continued dissatisfaction in the Kazak areas was the settlement of Han Chinese in northern Xinjiang. Migration was heavy in the 1950s, and it continued even in the difficult years of 1959–1961. Based on the increased populations of many towns and cities in central Xinjiang, a large number of migrants were sent to places like Shihezi and Wusu; the oil fields of Karamai, northwest of Urumqi also received permanent Han settlers. Others were sent to the PCC enterprises and to the new state farms, some of which were established on former Kazak grazing lands.

The activities of the PCC in the 1950s and 1960s were of great economic import. More than any other institution or organization, the PCC transformed the economic base in Xinjiang. By 1960, it had 182 state farms; and by 1961 it cultivated on vast mechanized farms fully one-third of the region's arable land. By 1965, the corps had reclaimed more than 10 million mu of land.[67] Maps showing the exact location of these enterprises during those years are not available. However, maps of such enterprises in the 1980s show many farms in the Tian Shan in central Xinjiang, in the northern districts of Tacheng and Altai, and along the major transport artery that runs westward from Hami through the regional capital, Urumqi, and to the Soviet border. PCC growth continued after a slowdown during the Cultural Revolution, when many of the Han assigned to Xinjiang were caught up in the turmoil of those years. By 1984, the PCC accounted for one-fourth of the autonomous region's total output of industrial and agricultural production, and it employed over 1 million people. In addition to the state farms, which were reduced in number to 169 by 1984, the PCC continued to run 729 industrial enterprises.[68] Other enterprises were developed in the southern part of the region, but PCC units continued to dominate the economy north of the Tian Shan.

Opposition to the PCC and its increasing share of the economy began early. In 1958, the government issued a vehement defense of the PCC's contribution to Xinjiang in the local press, in an attempt to counter criticism:

> The opposition to the PCC in Xinjiang Military District is the most outstanding expression of the opposition to the Han people engaging in socialist construction in Xinjiang, for most of the participants are Han people. . . . Some people may say that they do not oppose or attack the PCC itself, but oppose and attack its mistakes and short-comings. If they really do so, they are doing a good thing. But the local nationalists do not do so at all. They do not love the PCC but attack it. They oppose the PLA and the Han people engaging in socialist construction in Xinjiang.[69]

Opposition to the increasing numbers of Han and to the PCC was not stilled. Government reports continued to defend the PCC and the policy of sending Han to the area in order to speed its development into a modern region. Xinjiang's "backward" economy and cultural conditions required the assistance of the more advanced Han, according to repeated stories in the local media. By 1965 the number of Han in the region had dramatically increased; a year later they would be joined by more radical arrivals, sent to lead the region in China's newest campaign—the Great Proletarian Cultural Revolution.

The Cultural Revolution in Kazak Areas

Details of the impact of the Cultural Revolution on Xinjiang's Kazaks are given in chapter 5, where the history of each autonomous Kazak area is recounted in more detail. Generally, this was a very difficult time for all Kazaks—but it was particularly bad for Kazaks who had joined the party or had publicly expressed their support for the party's goals. Kazaks who joined the Red Guards later recounted stories of having to forcibly reeducate older Kazaks, burn their traditional-style clothes, cut off the men's beards and mustaches, and otherwise insult respected Kazak elders. A popular, possibly apocryphal story of this period is of an elderly Kazak who was praying at home when his young grandson entered the room. The boy shouted, "A thousand years of life to Chairman Mao," echoing the slogans of the Red Guards. The man hit his grandson to stop him from spoiling his prayers. Angered, the boy ran outside and told the Red Guards his grandfather had hit him for praising Mao. When the Guards stormed into the house to punish the old man, the Kazak said, "I was praying to Allah, asking him to give Chairman Mao ten thousand years of life when that stupid boy rushed in and started shouting 'One thousand years to Mao!' I thought that one thousand years was not sufficient for our Chairman and that is why I hit him."[70]

Like their Han Chinese counterparts, Kazak cadre also disappeared during this time, caught up in the machinations of contending factions within the party. Kazaks were persecuted under various pretexts, according to a Hui official interviewed in Xinjiang in 1983. Some were labeled "local nationalists" and were accused of having secret relations with foreign countries, particularly with the Kazak Soviet Socialist Republic. A number of Kazak cadres were jailed on the basis of such accusations.[71]

A major indicator of the impact of the Cultural Revolution in Kazak areas is the dramatic drop in the number of animals in the Ili-Kazak Autonomous Prefecture, which lost 30 percent of its animals.[72] Overall, herd numbers did not recover until 1982 (see table 5.7). Agriculture production also fell in Kazak areas, regaining pre–Cultural Revolution levels only in the early 1980s.[73]

An unanswered question arising from the decade-long Cultural Revolution is the extent of the movement's influence on the rise of what the Chinese term "local nationalism" among Xinjiang's Kazaks. Always deemed the major danger facing the northwest, any expression of nationalism among the region's ethnic minorities provided justification for the detention and arrest of minorities throughout the area. Reports in the Chinese press referred obliquely to underground nationalist organizations, shadowy entities funded by shadowy individuals somewhere outside the region. Given Xinjiang's history, the existence of such groups during the Cultural Revolution is likely enough; but, ironically, rumors of the existence of these groups probably helped the Chinese maintain tight control far more than the actual organizations ever aided Kazaks in their opposition to the Chinese and their policies. Whether this remains the case in the 1990s is unclear.

Kazak Areas in the Reform Era, 1978–1996

The death of Mao and the rise of Deng Xiaoping brought changes that were viewed positively by the Kazaks and other Muslims in Xinjiang. Attempts were made to heal the wounds of the Cultural Revolution, with Kazak and other minority cadre exonerated and restored to party membership and posts. Kazaks, along with other Muslims and many Han Chinese, were released from prisons and camps. Mosques resumed religious services, and restrictions on cultural activities relaxed. The previously banned Arabic script was reintroduced, and publications in the Kazak language grew in number and availability.

Following the Cultural Revolution, the administration of Kazak areas returned to the system that called for proportionate representation in autonomous governments for all resident nationalities. Had this been strictly applied after 1976, however, the Kazaks would barely have had a voice in any area of Xinjiang after 1980, for they no longer constituted a majority in any of the Kazak autonomous areas. In what can only be viewed as an attempt to continue the fiction of a functional autonomous system in Xinjiang, the percentage of Kazaks in local people's congresses was kept high, quite out of proportion to their numbers. In the early 1980s, of the total 555 seats in the Ili-Kazak people's congress, for example, Kazaks held 40 percent of the seats, although they only accounted for 24 percent of the prefecture's total population. On the more powerful standing committee of the congress they held 39 percent of the 43 seats. Similar patterns could be seen in the other Kazak areas of Mori and Barkol (see chapter 5).

As real power remained in party hands, the number of Kazaks in the

CCP provides a better indication both of Kazak power in local government and of their willingness to participate in government and local administration following the Cultural Revolution. As noted previously, the number of minority cadre in the CCP declined during the turbulent years from 1966 to 1976. Beginning in 1978, the party recruited actively to rebuild the shattered membership. As a result, the number of Kazak party members grew slowly in the 1980s. In 1982, the Ili-Kazak Autonomous Prefecture reported 21,796 Kazak cadre out of a total of 78,002. Of the Kazak cadre, 18,171 were also members of the Communist Party.[74]

By the 1990s, the party apparatus in all the Kazak areas nonetheless remained largely Han-dominated. In 1994, the party secretary of the Ili-Kazak prefecture was a Han, with two Kazaks serving as vice-secretaries along with one Han and one Uyghur. The CPPCC (Chinese People's Political Consultative Congress) was also chaired by a Han, supported by two Han vice-chairmen, two Kazak and two Uyghur vice-chairman, and one Mongol. Of all the party and government posts, only the position of *zhouzhang,* or prefectural chairman, continued to be a Kazak.

One of the two highest-ranking Kazaks in the Xinjiang political system was Beg Mehmet Musa (Biekemuhamaiti Musa), who was named head of the Ili-Kazak prefecture in 1994. Serving as his vice-chairmen are two Han Chinese, two Kazaks, and one Uyghur.[75] Higher ranked was Janabil, a Kazak who became a regional vice-secretary of the Xinjiang CCP in 1992. According to the Chinese media, Janabil, who was born in 1934, has been a party member since 1953, holding a variety of party posts in Konghe county, the Altay district, and the Ili-Kazak prefecture. A college graduate, he remained the senior Kazak representative in the CCP in 1996.

Although a few Kazaks expressed satisfaction with a policy that placed Kazaks at the head of local autonomous governments and in selected party posts, a new policy in 1996 regarding assignment of posts by ethnicity met with some resistance. In May of that year, the government announced that all village heads were to be Han. As this is the one official with whom most local people would have to deal regularly, this arbitrary change in policy was very unpopular and may have contributed to increasing tensions in the Yining area.

Another unwelcome aspect of Chinese policy since 1978 has been the continuation and expansion of *laogai* (reform through labor) camps and prisons throughout Xinjiang. Historically, the region had been a place of punishment, where erring officials and condemned criminals were sent under the sentence of banishment. The last dynasty continued this tradition, sending into exile in Xinjiang such notables as Commissioner Lin Zexu, the principal figure in the nineteenth-century Opium War.[76] In the early twentieth century, prison conditions in the region were notorious, with inmates dying as a result of appalling deprivation. Victims included both Han Chinese as well as Muslims. Those who emerged bore the scars of their incarceration in the form of physical illnesses like tuberculosis or mental distress.

Under the PRC, Xinjiang has been the site of both new laogai camps, which are primarily for political prisoners, and ordinary prisons for criminals. Relatively little is known about either type of facility or about the ethnic composition of those interned. The Laogai Research Foundation in the United States asserts that Xinjiang has at least fifteen laogai camps and three prisons, each with 2,000 to 10,000 prisoners—in addition to an unknown number of detention centers. The PCC reportedly uses laogai labor in six of its ten agricultural divisions in Xinjiang. The Chinese authorities do not release information on the identity, location, or number of those held in these facilities, but émigré Kazaks and Uyghurs believe many Muslims are held in this Chinese "gulag" system.

In the post–Cultural Revolution era, however, the most significant changes have concerned neither political reform nor the penal system; rather, it has been the series of important economic changes beginning in 1978 that has had the greatest impact on the Kazaks—as on all peoples in Xinjiang. The communes were eliminated in the region (a process described in more detail in chapters 5 and 6), and Kazaks regained control of their herds. "Free" markets allowed Kazaks to sell animals, meat, and hides for the best price they could get, although the return to herd ownership also brought a new system of grassland and slaughter taxes—among other monetary levies—on all pastoralists. Kazaks prospered as the economy improved, and per capita rural income increased overall to around 1,000 yuan annually by 1994.[77]

Kazaks also benefited by the expansion of tourism in Xinjiang after 1978. In that year, Xinjiang had a total of 88 foreign tourists; but ten years later, in 1987, the region welcomed 50,000.[78] By 1994, the total number of overseas tourists was 160,000.[79] Many of this number were members of escorted tours, moving along the Silk Road and visiting ancient sites that had been renovated, repaired, and restored throughout the 1980s with government funds. A growing number of independent travelers also visited the region, and most restrictions on previously closed areas were lifted.

In the 1980s, Kazaks who had camped for the summer at Tianchi Lake—a four- to five-hour bus ride from Urumqi—began renting horses for ten yuan a day to young travelers who wanted a memorable experience "among the nomads." By 1986, tourist cabins were available on the lake's shore, competing with Kazak yurts where travelers could spend the night with the family, sharing their food and quilts.

Traditionally, Kazaks welcomed any traveler to stop and visit, to drink salted milk-tea, and to share the family's meal and, if needed, accommodation. Charging for this traditional welcome has now become commonplace in Kazak areas near cities like Urumqi. One explanation offered for this is that some years ago Han began to visit the Kazak areas in the summer to escape the heat of the cities; they were welcomed in the traditional way, without any expectation of payment. However, when Kazaks went to Urumqi to visit, they anticipated reciprocal treatment and were affronted when it was not forthcoming. As a result, they began to charge for the food and accommodation that had been offered freely only a few years before. Whatever the motivation or its sources, the practice in 1996 was to charge for all services provided by Kazaks on grasslands near the regional capital.

The increase in foreign visitors has made visits to Kazak areas a part of the regular tourist circuit. Visitors can stay the night in an "authentic" yurt, now conveniently built on a permanent but definitely not traditional cement base, with amenities such as bottled gas stoves for cooking, electric lights, tape decks, and privacy (the family moves out temporarily) for only two hundred yuan. Tours of the grasslands at Nanshan, famous for its waterfall at the head of its long valley, are available by horse-drawn cart. The more adventurous can rent a horse, complete with a Kazak child on the back to make sure that an inexperienced rider will not harm himself—or the horse.

By 1996, the government-run China Travel Service competed with young Kazaks who, armed with their own name cards identifying them as representatives of what usually turned out to be one- or two-man operations, sought business in front of tourist hotels. Rather than allowing all the money being made on tourism in Kazak areas to fall into

Chinese hands, these entrepreneurs offered English-speaking tour guides for independent, budget-conscious travelers. Although such income is seasonal, it has the added attraction of allowing this enterprising group of young Kazaks to practice their English and Chinese, even as they carve out a Kazak presence in the informal tourist industry in Xinjiang.

While the Kazaks have generally experienced an increase in income following the economic reforms, and while some enterprising individuals have done quite well for themselves, overall the increases for Kazaks lag well behind that of Han Chinese—increasing Kazak concerns over the continued arrival of Han Chinese in the region. Some new Han arrivals still join the predominantly Han PCC, which has continued to expand its operations. In particular, its animal husbandry operations have drawn Kazak resentment, as have PCC efforts to attract more Han to Xinjiang. For instance, in 1996, some 20,000 migrant Han were farming land recently contracted from the Xinjiang Tianshan Nanbei Military Corps. Workers from Sichuan reportedly made an average of 4,200 yuan a year beginning in 1994, an extremely high salary. In 1995 alone, a few workers reportedly earned 170,000 yuan, a fortune for a Chinese peasant farmer.[80] Whether such stories were true or not, the broadcasting of such tales has no doubt served to fuel further Han movement into the northwest.

In the 1990s the Han presence in Kazak areas was being felt acutely. Already in the middle of the 1980s, reports of public demonstrations and protests in Kazak areas began to appear in the local media, with the intensity escalating in the 1990s. As will be discussed in chapter 6, the most violent of these occurred in the Ili area in 1995 and again in 1997. Primarily spontaneous outbursts, these violent episodes were set off in both years by what was locally perceived as interference in Muslim religious practices. The volatile situation will doubtless continue as long as the primary sources of complaint continue; indeed, the situation may be exacerbated by the activities of Kazaks just across the border in the new Republic of Kazakstan, a topic to which we return in chapter 7.

— 5 —

Life at the Local Level: Development and Change in Xinjiang's Autonomous Kazak Areas

In 1984 and 1985, official accounts of each of the Xinjiang-Uyghur Autonomous Region's three largest autonomous Kazak areas appeared in Urumqi bookstores, providing brief official histories and general overviews of cultural and economic development since 1949. As evinced by each book's appended *dashi nianbiao,* giving a chronology of significant events from the third century B.C. through the early 1980s, these small volumes were intended not only to provide Chinese readers with an understanding of the Kazak areas of Xinjiang, but also to illustrate these areas' historical development as parts of China. By linking the Kazak past with that of the Chinese empire, the present government conveys its message of historical Chinese sovereignty over the northwest and offers an implicit justification for continued Chinese governance there.

In this chapter, we focus separately on each of the three Kazak areas: the Ili-Kazak Autonomous Prefecture, the Barkol-Kazak Autonomous County, and the Mori-Kazak Autonomous County. This is for several reasons. First, we want to examine—as far as our sources allow—whether there have been significant differences in the experiences of Kazaks in the three subregional areas since 1949. Given subregional variations in topography, population density, ethnic composition, and economic development, one would expect such differences; and material presented in this chapter indeed suggests that each Kazak subregion is distinct both in terms of Chinese policy implementation and Kazak response.

In this regard, it is worth noting that in much of the recent literature on minorities—whether published in China or in the West—individual minority groups are often presented as though they constitute single, unified entities; and by implication they are possessed of a unified response to Chinese policy. As more information has become available, however, it has become clear that such an image is misleading. Indeed, recent research on minorities and minority areas shows a range of responses, varying along a broad continuum. Studying Xinjiang's three Kazak areas allows us to examine this varied response in more detail.

The three case studies also allow closer examination of important aspects of Han-Kazak interaction at the local level. We would like to know, for instance, whether initial policy implementation was flexible in accommodating the differing histories of the three areas. What was the nature of ethnic interaction in 1949, and how have shifts in the ethnic composition of these areas influenced such relations? Has the impact of Han migration in the three areas varied, or is there a relatively uniform response to the post-1949 demographic changes? What accommodations are both ethnic groups making in light of continued central government support of Han enterprises in Xinjiang's Kazak areas? And to what extent are economic reforms influencing ethnic relations—for better or for worse? The county and prefectural levels allow closer examination of the still-difficult terrain of interethnic relations, both between Han and Kazak and between Kazak and other minorities.

Sources remain problematic for the study of these and other subregional units in China, however. As we have noted, Chinese-language sources have their own political agendas, portraying the past and present in the light best suited to current government political objectives. Agendas aside, sanctioned Chinese accounts of Xinjiang Kazak areas are nonetheless an important source for the official state and party view of Kazak history and status. Also, while the statistics contained in these and other PRC sources may not have the degree of accuracy demanded in the West, they cannot be discounted, particularly insofar as they do not present a uniformly flattering picture of policy outcomes since 1949.

In addition to Chinese-language sources, the three case studies also draw upon interviews with Kazaks and other Muslims from Xinjiang. We also have used the small number of Western anthropological stud-

Table 5.1

Ethnic Distribution in the Ili-Kazak AP's Three Districts, 1990

Area	Total Population	Uyghur	Han	Kazak
Ili	1,819,575	503,114	586,721	413,635
Tacheng	777,414	36,539	445,339	197,113
Altay	511,689	10,666	216,645	255,598

Source: FBIS-CHI–90–250 (December 28, 1990), 55.

ies of Kazaks completed since 1980 and a wide variety of secondary sources. Together, these sources suggest that while there are overall patterns discernible in Kazak participation in post-1949 political and economic changes and in interethnic relations, the variations in each subregion's ethnic composition, percentage of urban population, level of economic development, and other factors have all influenced the relative status of Kazaks at the autonomous county and prefectural levels.

Ili-Kazak Autonomous Prefecture

The Ili-Kazak Autonomous Prefecture (Yili Hasake zizhizhou) was officially founded on November 28, 1954, the last of the three subregional Kazak areas to be established in Xinjiang. It is the largest and most important Kazak unit, both in population and area, and is the only prefecture-level governmental unit for Kazaks in China.

The prefecture covers 267,400 square kilometers, and in 1994 it had a total population of 3.55 million, a quarter of which was Kazak. As in other parts of Xinjiang, the single most important demographic change since 1949 has been the arrival of large numbers of Han Chinese, both civilian and military (see figures in tables 5.1 and 5.2). Official population figures do not include the Han serving in units of the PCC, nor do they include men in the military units assigned to this key border area. Excluding these groups, the Han Chinese population in 1994 was 1,570,000, or 44.2 percent of the prefecture's inhabitants, which is up 10 percent over figures for 1991. The Ili prefecture's minority population, which totaled 1,976,000 in 1994, included 934,000 Kazaks (26.3 percent of the prefecture's inhabitants) and 568,000 Uyghurs (16 per-

Table 5.2

Ili-Kazak Autonomous Prefecture's Population Growth by Nationality

Nationality	1944	1982	1991	1994
Kazak	383,569	709,500	896,140	934,000
Uyghur	90,222	470,700	549,874	568,000
Han	57,994	1,393,500	1,491,398	1,570,000
Hui	—	211,800	270,425	—
Kirghiz	—	12,700	15,651	—
Mongol	43,164	52,100	61,907	—
Xibo	—	25,184	30,116	—
Russian	—	1,600	4,108	—
Tajik	—	300	113	—
Uzbek	—	5,600	4,675	—
Tatar	—	2,500	2,518	
Manchu	—	2,600	3,639	—
Daur	—	4,100	4,961	—
Other	184,348	40,800	48,166	477,000
Total	759,297	2,933,500	3,383,691	3,549,000

Sources: The 1944 figures are from *Tianshan yuegan* (October 15, 1947), 10–13. The 1982 figures are from *Yili Hasake zizhizhou gaikuang,* 13. The actual total is 2,932,984 rather than the 2,933,500 given in the original source. (No explanation is given in the 1991 source for the drop in the number of Tajiks.) The 1991 figures are from *Xinjiang nianjian 1992.* The 1994 figures are from *Xinjiang nianjian 1995,* and according to the source does not include members of the PCC.

cent). The remaining 477,000 (13.4 percent) are members of other nationalities.[1] The prefectural capital is Yining, 702 kilometers from Urumqi; its population in 1991 was 267,000, of which only 12,000 (4 percent) were Kazak. Like other urban areas, the prefectural capital has a large Han population, over 85,000 (32 percent). Uyghurs constitute the majority at 51 percent of the population, or over 137,000, in 1991.[2] The prefectural capital's population rose to 289,775 in 1994, but no breakdown by ethnic group is provided for that year. Figures on the growth of Xinjiang's largest cities are given in table 5.3.

The Ili-Kazak Autonomous Prefecture has three districts under its administration: these are Ili, Tacheng, and Altay, which together comprised the East Turkestan Republic of 1944–1950. However, within each of the districts there are also autonomous counties for other nationalities, so that the contemporary political configuration does not

Table 5.3

Growth in Xinjiang Urban Populations

City	Years	Total Population	Minority Population
Yining	1982	220,000	—
	1991	267,262	181,444
	1994	289,775	190,163
Kuitun	1982	50,000	—
	1994	90,121	6,362
Tacheng	1982	37,000	—
	1991	131,238	47,216
	1994	138,492	49,365
Altay	1982	34,000	—
	1991	183,567	74,158
	1994	166,300	75,700
Shihezi	1964	70,000	—
	1991	533,710	24,002
Karamay	1959	50,000	—
	1991	210,208	50,514
Urumqi	1949	80,000	—
	1981	850,000	—
	1989	1,200,000	312,000
Hami	1991	1,336,456	362,424
	1994	314,334	103,779

Sources: Figures are taken from *Yili-Hasake zizhizhou gaikuang* (1985); *Balikun-Hasake zizhixian gaikuang* (1984); and *Mulei-Hasake zizhixian gaikuang* (1984). Figures for the 1990s, which do not include workers, are from various editions of *Xinjiang nianjian.*

replicate that of the 1940s. Of the twenty counties in the prefecture, two are autonomous: the Chapchal Xibo Autonomous County under the Ili district, created for the Manchu-speaking Xibo minority; and the Hoboksar (Hebukesaier) Mongol Autonomous County in the Tacheng district. In addition to the autonomous counties, the relatively new boomtown of Kuitun is directly under prefectural control. Three other urban areas are also classified as cities: the district capitals of Tacheng and Altay as well as the prefectural capital, Yining (see table 5.4 for

Table 5.4

Population Growth in the Ili-Kazak Autonomous Prefecture by District

Area	1944	1991	1994
Yining	505,035	1,834,463	1,929,214
Tacheng	170,422	798,701	770,763
Altay (Ashan)	83,840	523,978	541,368

Sources: The 1944 figures are from *Tianshan yuegan* (October 15, 1947), 10–13. The 1991 figures are from *Xinjiang nianjian 1992,* 40. The 1994 figures are from *Xinjiang nianjian 1995,* 400, 411, 420.

population growth in the three districts of the Ili-Kazak Autonomous Prefecture).

The Ili prefecture's geographical location has determined its recent political history. It lies in a strategic position along China's western border, a border previously shared with the USSR but, since 1991, with the Republic of Kazakstan. In the nineteenth century the prefecture's three districts became a buffer separating the imperial Russian and Chinese states, making it an element in what was romantically referred to as the "Great Game," a contest for power and influence between Great Britain, Imperial Russia, and the Qing dynasty. Although the area was claimed by the Qing court and Chinese troops were stationed there beginning in the eighteenth century, rebellions against Qing rule punctuated the region's history, culminating in the rebellion of Yakub Beg, who declared himself ruler of an independent state that extended from his base at Kashgar to all the cities of the Tarim Basin and the lands north of the Tian Shan by 1870. Although the Qing were able to defeat Yakub Beg's forces in 1877, Russia took the opportunity afforded by turmoil in the region to occupy the fertile Ili River valley in the 1870s, returning it only after intense diplomatic negotiations in 1881. It was after this incident, in 1884, that the Qing formally declared all of the northwestern territory to be a province for the first time in Chinese history.

In addition to its strategic location, the Ili area was also desirable for its agriculture and animal husbandry. Blessed with the highest precipitation in Xinjiang, the Ili Valley is also shielded from the region's harsh winters by two branches of the Tian Shan that converge to the east. The valley produces an abundance of fruit and grains, and mountain pastures to the north and south provide summer grazing for herds that shelter in the valleys during the winter months.

As in the past, forests remain a major resource today, covering 497,333 hectares and providing a protected habitat for many wild animals, including sable, silver fox, red deer, over twenty species of fish, and many rare birds. The valley is famous for the Ili horse, prized by Chinese armies for centuries and still bred for export as well as local use.

Potential for industrial development was recognized at the end of the nineteenth century, when early explorers from the West began reporting on the mineral wealth of the area. Among other ores, the autonomous prefecture has coal, iron, gold, silver, and uranium.

In the twentieth century, the prefecture's population shared the fortunes of the rest of Xinjiang, which have been described earlier in this book. It was recognized internationally as a part of China after the 1912 revolution; but local nationalists, influenced by pan-Turkic and pan-Islamic movements as well as by nationalism and republicanism, were not daunted by that recognition and continued to advocate not only an independent Ili area but an independent East Turkestan, comprising all of Xinjiang Province. The warlords who ruled Xinjiang from 1912 until 1944 continued to face the challenge of indigenous demands for autonomy and independence. The Ili River valley served as the headquarters for the last East Turkestani republican movement, and was independent of Nationalist Chinese control from 1944 to 1949. Thus the one single area in Xinjiang of greatest concern to the CCP and the newly arrived PLA in 1949–1950 was the highly sensitive Ili area and its allied districts of Tacheng and Altay.

It is not surprising, therefore, that the CCP moved cautiously at first, concentrating on the district's farming areas, where peasants constituted a familiar focus for CCP activities. However, the less accessible Kazaks, many of whom remained armed, required a different approach. While the CCP grappled with the issue of what policy to pursue in the Kazak areas, they prepared the ground in settled areas for the CCP message.

One means by which to accomplish this was to show respect for the still-popular East Turkestani government and its leaders. Possibly at the urging of Saifudin, a well-publicized memorial meeting for the East Turkestan's deceased leaders was held in November 1949, even before the CCP had arrived in force in the area. The following year,

the local press again featured coverage of memorial services, emphasizing the roles of Ahmetjan Kasimi, who was born near Yining, and
Ishak Han Mura Haji, the Kirghiz leader from the Ili area. Services
were attended by important Han and minority leaders from all over
Xinjiang.

In addition to honoring popular past leaders, the government also
used the opportunity afforded by such services to remind the people of
the oppression they had suffered under Guomindang-affiliated warlords like Yang, Jin, and Sheng Shicai. The latter, in particular, was
singled out in the press as responsible for the deaths of many important
individuals from the Ili area; it was to overthrow such tyrants that the
people had joined the East Turkestani republican movement. Another
common enemy identified in such stories was Osman Batur, who became a useful figure to the new government as it attempted to unite the
people politically through their own troubled, shared past—a continuing theme in 1990s publications as well.[3]

The arrival of CCP cadre and the PLA in the three districts during
the winter of 1949–1950 began a period characterized in Chinese
sources as a time of great struggle to raise the political consciousness
of the local population. Although PRC publications on this period
acknowledge the revolutionary nature of the East Turkestan Republic,
the actions of the party and the PLA in their first two years in Ili
suggest that in fact they were unconvinced there was any real local
commitment to communism. Thus, despite the CCP's proclamation
that the Three Districts Revolution was a part of the whole Chinese
people's revolution, the new government chose not to rely on local
leaders to establish a new socialist order in Xinjiang. Instead, they
assigned 1,000 army cadre under the leadership of a Han Chinese,
Ceng Di, for this important and sensitive work.

The initial focus was on agricultural rather than pastoral areas.
Work began with meetings to explain the new religious policy, the
guarantees of equality, and the ways in which the local people should
oppose "feudalism." The latter became the basis for a struggle against
the local landlords, 4.6 percent of whom held 31 percent of the land,
according to CCP reports.[4] Only 15 percent of villagers had their own
land, while 52 percent of all villagers were classified as "poor peasants" and "farm laborers."[5] Work in farming areas thus focused on rent
reduction and "opposition to local despots"—themes that were being
followed elsewhere in China. Efforts intensified in 1952, when 82,000

people reportedly attended meetings to raise political consciousness. Despite such impressive numbers and optimistic government depictions of the situation in Ili, Kazak resistance continued in 1950–1952. PLA units were assigned the task of suppressing this opposition. Assisting them were former members of the East Turkestani military, which, in 1949–1950, had been incorporated into the PLA as the new Fifth Army. Osman's defection from the republic and his subsequent attacks on the Altay area in 1947 may have made his pursuit a welcome assignment for the men of the new Fifth Army.[6]

The life of the new Fifth Army, however, was short. In the early 1950s, many units were reorganized and then reassigned outside the Ili area. An undisclosed number of former East Turkestani officers were sent to Beijing and other cities in eastern China for training, effectively removing potentially troublesome republican military leaders from Xinjiang. The Fifth Army itself was dissolved abruptly in 1954, in circumstances that remain unclear.

As the PLA consolidated its control in the towns and villages, CCP cadre began working to establish lower-level governments, bringing Kazaks into the process as far as possible. In 1951, local representatives were appointed to a people's representatives congress (*Renmin daibiao hui*), which in turn arranged the prefecture's first people's congress (*Renmin daibiao dahui*) convened the following year. As table 5.5 shows, the prefecture's 1952 congress was composed of 271 representatives, including 138 Kazaks, or 51 percent of the total.

By 1954, the government considered the three districts to be securely under PLA and CCP control. Thus the Ili-Kazak Autonomous Prefecture was formally established in November 1954, and its government was given powers and responsibilities in accord with the guidelines for minority areas provided in China's 1954 constitution. With the prefectural government in place, efforts to move the area forward on the "socialist road" began in earnest.

The economic reorganization of the prefecture's pastoral areas was the focus of discussion at the 1954 Second Pastoral Districts Work Meeting in Urumqi, following which the Ili prefecture initiated major economic changes, beginning with a call to form mutual-aid teams. Over the next two years, work continued on this project, resulting, by the spring of 1956, in the formation of 2,300 mutual-aid teams among the herding population. While the number seemed impressive, the teams incorporated only one-third of the region's herders, indicating

Table 5.5

1952 Ili-Kazak Autonomous Prefecture People's Congress

Nationality	1952 Number	%	1983 Number	%
Kazak	138	50.9	226	41
Uyghur	71	26.2	—	—
Han	20	7.4	—	—
Hui	11	4.0	—	—
Mongol	10	3.7	—	—
Xibo	5	1.8	—	—
Tatar	4	1.5	—	—
Kirghiz	3	1.1	—	—
Uzbek	3	1.1	—	—
Russian	3	1.1	1	0.2
Daur	2	0.7	1	0.2
Manchu	1	0.4	1	0.2
Total	271	99.9	555	

Source: Figures are from *Yili Hasake zizhizhou gaikuang,* 63–64.

that party efforts had limited success. Nonetheless, a year later, in 1957, the prefecture was urged to move its mutual-aid teams up a level, to that of the herder cooperatives. In response, 558 of these new economic units formed, accounting for 40.5 percent of the area's herders. A further push in 1958 resulted in a total of 939 co-ops which reportedly included 71.5 percent of the district's animal herding families.[7]

While considerable headway had been made in directing the Ili economy down the socialist road by 1958, it lagged behind the rest of China. In herding areas in particular, local authorities tolerated a slower rate of change, reflecting both early Kazak resistance and continued reluctance to change traditional practices. Chinese press reports indicate that as late as 1958 there was still private herd-ownership in one form or another. For example, in 1958 the media reported a total of fifty-nine "state-private" co-ops in the Ili prefecture. Herd owners received interest payments of 2–4 percent, based on the number of animals they contributed to the co-op herd. While the appearance of purely private ownership of herds was avoided, individual herd owners nonetheless effectively retained ownership of their herds.

Despite the relatively slow pace of change, unrest continued. In the charged atmosphere of the Anti-Rightist campaign during the summer of 1957, there were "disturbances" in Yining, reportedly caused by "various types of enemies," including convicts from laogai camps in the Ili prefecture.[8] When the results of the trials for these counterrevolutionaries and other "bad elements" appeared in the press, only Chinese names were listed, suggesting that this first incident was a part of the local political struggle associated with the Anti-Rightist campaign.

In late November 1957, the local press reported demands that clearly originated with the area's Kazaks and Uyghurs. These included a call for the formation of a new Eastern Turkestan, in which Uyghurs and Kazaks would rule the Xinjiang region independently. Another demand was for the establishment of the Communist Party locally on national lines, making local party officials accountable in Xinjiang not Beijing. In what would become a feature of all demonstrations and lists of grievances against the Han-led government from them on, local Muslims also called for the expulsion of Han cadres and all Han settlers from Xinjiang. Kazak officials' obligatory public denunciation of these demands had little impact. The government's response became clear by the end of the year when a new harsher line began to take effect.

A significant aspect of this new line was the purge of minority leaders that took place the following year. The most prominent of those purged was Yahuda, the Kazak chairman of the prefecture, who was ousted in 1958 despite his vigorous denunciation of local national-ists the previous year.[9]

The CCP also curtailed public observance of religious festivals and celebrations. Beginning in 1957 and continuing through 1962, refer-ences in the press to religious holidays for Ramadan and Kurban-bairam disappeared. Activities of the officially sanctioned Muslim association were also curtailed, as was permission for Muslims to travel to Mecca on hajj.

In January 1959, a further indication that the central government was now requiring local conformity to national policies came in the form of revisions to Xinjiang's marriage regulations. Under the auton-omy system, the autonomous region was empowered to pass laws in keeping with local conditions; accordingly, it had allowed marriages at somewhat earlier ages than was permitted elsewhere in China. Now, however, the marriage age was raised from eighteen to twenty for men and from sixteen to eighteen for women, in conformity to national standards.[10]

As in other parts of China, the years between 1958 and 1962 were difficult, marked by food shortages and tightened government control.

In minority areas like Ili, economic difficulties caused by the Great Leap Forward were exacerbated by the new crackdown on Muslim practices and the required conformity to nationally mandated policies. Predictably, discontent increased. Unlike other parts of China, however, the Ili prefecture's location on the Soviet border provided an option not available elsewhere. In 1962 thousands chose to leave Ili for the neighboring Kazak Soviet Socialist Republic.

In Xinjiang this exodus is referred to as the Yi-Ta incident, so named for the Yili (Ili) and Tarbagatay areas from which the majority of refugees fled. Kazaks and Uyghurs, as well as other residents of the three districts who had retained one of the thousands of Soviet passports issued to Xinjiang residents in the 1930s and 1940s, began to leave in small numbers in the late 1950s. By 1962 deteriorating conditions led many to sell their houses and property and to move across the border in a mass exodus.

The flight of thousands of residents from Xinjiang was not reported in the Chinese media. It was not until 1964 that Premier Zhou Enlai referred to the incident briefly in a speech denouncing the USSR, noting only that thousands of people had left the region.[11] Later reports from China supplied little additional information.[12] Recent Chinese-language sources remain equally reticent, simply noting that as a result of foreign influence, several tens of thousands left in 1962, taking their livestock with them.[13]

Kazaks and other Muslims now living outside China are more forthcoming. They recall that in 1962, many thousands of Kazaks and Uyghurs holding Soviet passports left the Ili prefecture, at first unimpeded by border guards. In the Tarbagatay area, whole villages reportedly left en masse, choosing life in the USSR over continued deprivations in China.[14] Other former Xinjiang residents assert that not only villages but whole counties decamped to the Soviet Union.

Because of the large numbers involved, angry Chinese authorities abruptly announced their intent to close the border, leaving only three days in which to make arrangements and go. As the only affordable means of transport was the bus system, which was already booked for months in advance, the government announcement meant in effect that no more residents would be allowed to leave. Nevertheless, though unable to sell their houses or arrange transport at short notice, some took advantage of the three-day grace period, taking only the clothes on their backs.[15]

On May 29, 1962, demonstrators gathered in the downtown area of the prefectural capital of Yining to protest government attempts to halt the migrations. The government broke up the demonstration by shooting into the crowd, killing and wounding an unknown number of Kazaks and Uyghurs. This event is now known locally as the Five Twenty-nine incident, for the date on which it occurred. In June, attempting to prevent any further incidents or border crossings, the authorities created a buffer zone along the immediate border, bringing in reinforcements of Han Chinese troops as border guards.

The number of people who fled before the border was effectively closed in 1962 remains difficult to determine. According to the Soviet press, the Uyghur population in the USSR grew from 95,000 in 1959 to 173,000 in 1970, suggesting sizable in-migration. The Hui population also rose from 22,000 to 39,000 in the same period.[16] Uyghurs and Kazaks outside of China say that the number of emigrants could be as high as 900,000, citing inaccurate census data that undercounted both groups in 1953 for political reasons. While the most likely number is in the range of 100,000 to 200,000 people, the issue of how many fled the region during the "three bitter years" remains unresolved.

The poor conditions in Xinjiang were partly to blame for the 1960–1962 flight of Kazaks and Uyghurs, but the steady arrival of Han Chinese settlers was another important factor in growing Muslim discontent (see table 5.6). After 1949, Ili's Han population had grown steadily but slowly; in 1959 the railway line linking Lanzhou and Urumqi finally reached Xinjiang's eastern oasis towns, speeding the transfer of Han Chinese to the far northwest. That summer, the press reported that workers and peasants had been pouring into the region since March in response to requests from the autonomous region's government for more manpower. Some 100,000 Han arrived between March and October 1959.[17] Some of the new arrivals were assigned to work on Xinjiang's PCC farms and ranches, which were absorbing excess labor from coastal China. Thousands of young people from Shanghai settled on PCC farms, some of which were on former Kazak grazing lands.

The PCC was very active in the Ili Valley from 1962 onwards: These predominantly Han units established four ranches in the valley by August 1962 and, in addition, operated fourteen mechanized farms cultivating a total of 1.3 million mu by the end of the summer.[18] Expanding the activities of this paramilitary presence was clearly viewed as one means by which to better control the politically unreliable local Muslim population.

Table 5.6

Han Population Growth in Xinjiang and the Ili-Kazak Autonomous Prefecture

Year	XUAR	Ili-Kazak AP
1944	222,401	57,994
1953	300,000	—
1954	550,904	—
1965	1,396,000	—
1970	2,650,000	—
1974	3,200,000	—
1982	5,286,533	1,393,500
1990	—	1,248,705
1991	5,769,393	1,491,398
1994	—	1,570,000

Sources: 1944 figures are from the *Tianshan yuegan* (October 15, 1947), 10–13; figures for 1953 through 1984 are from *Xinjiang-Weiwuer zizhiqu gaikuang* (1985), 317; *Yili Hasake zizhizhou gaikuang* (1985), 13. The 1990 figures are from the 1992 and 1995 *Xinjiang nianjian.*

With order restored and the Han military strengthened by new reinforcements and the presence of an expanded PCC, the party set about mending ethnic relations, offering a respite from the more oppressive aspects of Chinese rule during the 1957–1962 period. The celebration of Muslim festivals, curtailed between 1957 and 1962 and not allowed at all in 1960, resumed, according to announcements in the local press. In the Ili-Kazak Autonomous Prefecture, the 1964 religious festivals were even marked with a three-day holiday and by heavy attendance at thirty mosques in Yining.[19] In Ili, as elsewhere in the region, cadre were cautioned to implement the party's religious policy correctly. Special foods and manufactured goods designed to minority tastes appeared in local markets: Lace veils and dresses, fur hats and boots, leather saddles and musical instruments produced in local workshops spoke of new tolerance for minority sensibilities. The head of the Ili-Kazak prefecture in 1965 was a Kazak, Irhali (Er-ha-li), and it appeared that the area would now prosper under his leadership.

In 1966 Chairman Mao launched the Cultural Revolution, beginning another difficult period for minorities all over China. Not surprisingly, this is a period on which PRC sources are relatively silent. The few, scattered reports and limited statistics available for this period paint a

Table 5.7

Animal Population, Ili-Kazak Autonomous Prefecture

Year	Number
1944	6,676,922
1949	3,070,000
1965	8,530,000
1975	7,352,000
1982	8,540,000
1994	103,996,000

Sources: The 1944 figure is from *Tianshan yuegan* (October 15, 1947), 10–13. The 1949–1982 figures are from *Yili Hasake zizhizhou gaikuang* (1985), 83. The 1994 figure is from *Xinjiang nianjian 1995,* 398.

dismal picture of life in the Kazak areas. One measure of the difficult conditions for Kazaks during this time are the numbers for animal populations, the traditional basis of the nomad economy. Officially, in the Ili prefecture alone, some 30 percent of all animals died in 1969. Some may have been killed by bad weather that year, others may have been moved by the Kazaks across the border to neighboring USSR or Mongolia. Whatever the causes, however, nearly one-third of the animals disappeared, and replacement of the herds was slow: As noted earlier, 1975 populations were still not up to the level of 1965 (see table 5.7).

The Cultural Revolution did not end because of the economic toll or because of the deterioration of ethnic relations in the Ili area. Rather, the central government was intimidated by violent border clashes with the USSR, near the town of Tacheng (Tarbagatay) in December 1968. Further clashes occurred to the north, on the Irtysh River, in May and June 1969.[20] In the face of this threat, the Cultural Revolution in Xinjiang officially ended in the summer of 1969, leaving the region's strongman, Wang Enmao, still in control of the regional government and party.

The early 1970s saw a new generation of Kazak cadre appointed to the regional government, to higher profile positions. Among these was Zuya, who was named as one of nine regional vice-chairmen and who, in 1973, was also appointed to the CCP's Central Committee.

By the end of the Cultural Revolution, the Ili-Kazak prefecture had changed in fundamental ways. One of the most significant changes

Table 5.8

Grain Production in the Ili-Kazak Autonomous Prefecture

Year	Amount (in Jin)
1949	340,000
1958	840,000
1966	1,300,000
1983	1,600,000
1994	2,647,820,000

Note: A jin equals 1/2 kilogram or 1.1 lb.

was in its ethnic composition: Han Chinese nearly equaled the Kazaks in number. Although Kazaks continued to have a substantial number of seats in the people's congresses at all levels, the numerical basis for sharing power equally with the Han Chinese was clearly in place by 1976.

The arrival of so many Han settlers also brought about another, probably irreversible change in land usage. The amount of agricultural land and grain production in the Ili prefecture increased steadily from 1958 onwards, reflecting land-reclamation efforts and higher productivity due to mechanization, as well as other improvements on state and PCC farms (see table 5.8). Overall, by the middle of the 1980s, 3.3 to 3.4 million hectares (50 million mu) of winter pasturage was converted to agricultural use throughout Xinjiang, much of it on the fringes of the Jungarian Basin. In addition, salinization and dessication affected another 4.7 million hectares (70 million mu), further decreasing the amount of land available to regional herds.[21]

The increasing acreage under cultivation may be one reason for the slow rate of growth in the animal population after the Cultural Revolution. Historically, the number of animals has always fallen during times of grave disturbance; thus, from 6.7 million in 1944 in Ili, the animal population fell to just over 3 million in 1949. By 1965, the number had recovered, exceeding 1944 levels at 8.5 million animals. After dropping during the Cultural Revolution, the number of animals again rose, reaching 7.4 million animals in 1975. That figure, however, was only about 700,000 over the 1944 figure. In 1982, the number rose to 8.5 million, back to the level of pre–Cultural Revolution days (see table 5.7 for animal populations).

In sum, by the time the Cultural Revolution officially ended in 1976, major changes had taken place in the Ili prefecture. First, the increased number of Han residing there made the Kazaks a numerical minority for the first time. Second, the increase in land under cultivation meant a concomitant decrease in grasslands available to animal herds. With fewer pastures and more demands on available water resources by the growing agricultural sector, further limitations were imposed on Kazaks wishing to practice a traditional nomadic lifestyle. These trends in population and land use have continued, and they remain the two most important aspects underlying the ongoing economic transformation of China begun during Deng Xiaoping's era of reform, to which we now turn.

Ili-Kazak Autonomous Prefecture in the Reform Era

The rise of Deng Xiaoping to political preeminence in 1978 began China's era of economic reform. The commune system was dismantled, replaced by the "contract responsibility system" under which peasants leased their land from the state and contracted to sell certain amounts to the state in return. Produce beyond the quota was sold on the private market. By the early 1980s, this system was instituted throughout China.

Xinjiang was among the last areas to begin economic reform, but by the mid-1980s, reforms had arrived. The following discussion focuses on some of the most important changes in the areas of agriculture, herding, income levels, and prefectural and regional government and party participation since 1980. Education, literacy, literature, and traditional cultural and religious practices are discussed in chapter 6; new trade relations with neighboring Kazakstan are discussed in chapter 7.

Agriculture

The government asserts that since 1958, grain output in the Ili-Kazak Autonomous Prefecture has increased 45 million kilograms a year. In addition, oil-bearing grains have increased 5 million kilograms in output. Such production is possible because of an increase in the number of agricultural workers—mainly Han Chinese settlers, who have worked diligently not only to grow food crops but also to reclaim land throughout the three districts of the Ili prefecture. In 1949, 4.3 million mu were cultivated in the prefecture, but by 1966 the total under cultivation reached 11 million mu. Productivity per mu also increased as greater efforts were put into the land, leading to the 1983 figure of 1.6 billion jin of grain harvested from the prefecture's fields. By 1994, 2.64 billion jin were harvested.[22]

The number of Kazaks directly involved in agricultural production is not known. A small number of Kazaks in the prefecture work on state and PCC farms, but the exact number who farm—or who combine farming with animal husbandry—is not available. The significance of the increase in agricultural production for the Kazaks lies in the amount of grassland diverted to this greatly expanded economic activity. PCC farms in the Ili River valley have incorporated former pasture lands, a pattern also seen in river valleys of the Tacheng and Altay districts to the north. In the Altay district, which still had a predominantly Kazak population in 1990 (255,000 Kazaks and 216,000 Han), there were only two PCC farms, suggesting a less intrusive role for the PCC. However, this may be less an indicator of Chinese desire to placate Kazaks than it is of the difficulties imposed by the distance of this area from the more populated areas of the autonomous region and by the lack of good roads or rail transportation.

The cultivation of land and the necessary diversion of water resources to supply the new farms and PCC enterprises have had an important impact on the staple of the Kazak traditional economy–animal husbandry. While animals and animal products remain a substantial part of the economy in the prefecture, it is likely that in the twenty-first century, manufacturing, exploitation of natural resources, and agriculture will dominate the economy—and the use of land resources in the prefecture. Family-run businesses relying on animal husbandry will become increasingly marginalized as the state farms and ranches increase their profits and their share of the market for animal products.

Animal Husbandry and Herding

Animals are the traditional basis of Kazak life, and thus the health and size of herds—of all kinds of animals but principally of sheep—have been traditional indicators of prosperity. In the reform era, herds have reverted to private ownership and are again the basis of family income.

But unlike the free economy of the pre-1949 period, the role of the state remains a key factor: Today the government controls access to land and water, sets prices for animal products, and, above all, continues its policy of eventually settling all herding families, ending transhumance as a way of life. This policy pits Han Chinese—in the government, on state and PCC farms, and in the military—firmly against those Kazaks who prefer to continue a nomadic lifestyle.

Since 1949, some groups of Kazaks have continued as nomads in the prefecture. Even after the establishment of the communes in 1958, Kazaks retained private ownership of a few animals, providing a link through the 1970s to the days of private herd ownership. The economic reforms of the last two decades have resulted in the dismantling of the herders' communes, once more allowing private ownership of herds. Commune animals were dispersed to individual families, leaving only the state-owned ranches' herds under government control.

The dissolution of the communes meant that animals in Kazak herds were of two kinds: Those that Kazak families owned as their private property and, on the other hand, those given to them as part of the division of former commune herds. Initially, the latter were still technically the property of the *xiang* (township), which replaced the commune. The family, however, was entitled to the usufruct of these animals, including sheeps' wool, milk, and lambs. The wool of the former commune sheep had to be sold to the government, as did some of the slaughtered animals; but apart from this, the family could dispose of their animals and animal products as they chose.[23]

In setting up the new system, the government allotted each family a portion of the animals from the commune herds; but some individuals no longer owned the equipment needed to continue or, in some cases, resume their life as herders. For instance, some Kazaks had accepted allotments of farmland and had turned to agriculture prior to the reforms.[24] Nonetheless, those Kazaks unable to return to herding accepted the animals allotted them, adding their animals to the herds of relatives. Arrangements for settling accounts include monetary payment.[25]

In 1986, the government moved to adjust what was still an ambiguous system of herd ownership. The value of the dispersed commune animals was fixed in monetary terms, and the herdsmen were told to pay that amount to the state over a ten- to fifteen-year period. As the original commune herds consisted of what originally were the Kazaks' own animals, they were, in effect, buying back their own livestock. These payments were in addition to the animal husbandry tax and a grasslands fee all herders owed to the state.[26] Further, the state required that 70 percent of the fleece be sold to the state, at state-fixed prices, with the remainder disposed of as the family chose.

As part of the new system, money paid to the state for use of the grasslands was to be invested in improvements to animal husbandry. This apparently did not occur, at least at the level expected. In 1990, Kazak prefectural officials voiced concerns that the central government had not paid adequate attention to development of pastoral areas. At the National People's Congress in 1990, representatives of China's pastoral areas complained that the government-work report circulated at the People's Congress neglected to even mention animal husbandry. Ashat, chairman of the Ili-Kazak prefecture and representative to the People's Congress, joined other representatives from pastoral areas in asking that the government implement new measures to expand animal husbandry. He proposed that pastureland development be placed under state planning because animal husbandry was not developing steadily. Chairman Ashat also gave several other reasons for the slow expansion of animal husbandry. These included poor capital construction, or, in other words, the lack of money invested in grassland management; "backward" culture—a phrase not explained in the report but presumably a reference to the lack of formal education among rural Kazaks and to their reluctance to change traditional aspects of life; and underdevelopment of the commodity economy in Xinjiang. Backing this request for greater government assistance was the assertion that without it, the political stability of the minority border areas would be affected.[27]

Following the collapse of the USSR in 1991 and the emergence of independent Kazakstan on the Ili-Kazak western border, the government clearly began to pay greater attention to minority border areas. In addition to encouraging border trade and allowing greater local autonomy in trade agreements, the central authorities also announced in 1995 a "new" mode of production for pastoral areas, combining natural grassland with man-made grassland for raising animals. Seasonal movement remained a part of the new method, with animals going out to pasture in the warm season and being fed in pens during the winter. Despite the upbeat tone of such reports, however, exact numbers of Kazaks attracted to the new methods were not given.[28]

The number of animals in the Ili prefecture had reached 8.5 million head in 1981. In 1994, the government reported a total animal population of nearly 104 million (see table 5.7).[29] Although the latter number is high, it includes both small animals—like pigs, which the Muslims do not raise—as well as larger animals like sheep and horses. The number is also problematic because it is not clear how many animals remain in state and PCC herds and how many are in privately owned herds.

Although the numbers of animals cited above is not very useful in determining who owns what and where, it is apparent that the core of CCP policy toward herding peoples like the Kazak remains the same as it has been since the 1950s: settle all Kazak herders. Chinese media has repeatedly stressed the successes enjoyed by those herdsmen who have chosen to follow CCP guidance and settle down. Only by settling down, the government reports stress, can herdsmen "shake off poverty."[30] However, even in the 1990s, news reports still referred to efforts that would "gradually help herdsmen to establish settlements or semi-settlements" indicating that a certain number of Kazaks continue their traditional nomadic lifestyle.[31]

Thus despite fifty years of state efforts, some Kazaks continue to defy the government, seemingly impervious to the blandishments of the CCP or the assurances that settling down would provide them with advantages such as schooling, medical care, and higher incomes. The change from communal ownership of herds to a private system in the middle of the 1980s has allowed some Kazaks to hold onto their traditional lifestyle, which will continue into the twenty-first century. However, the increasing levels of cultivated land, the growth of the Han Chinese farming population, and the PCC enterprises ensure that the opportunities to continue this lifestyle decrease with each passing year.

Interviews with Kazaks in 1996 indicated that while some young Kazaks are attracted to the possibilities provided by a settled lifestyle, Kazaks in the Altay and Tacheng districts wish to continue the old ways of living. Current policies of private, family ownership of herds encourage continuation of old patterns, albeit within limitations imposed by the growing agricultural sector. Further, as of 1996 it appeared that the government had postponed further efforts to settle Kazaks. Instead of pushing a still-resisted—and in some areas still-resented—policy, the government is relying on economic reforms and the continued policy of "opening up" Xinjiang to the outside world to bring about change among the prefecture's still-nomadic Kazaks. There is some evidence to suggest that Kazaks have begun taking advantage of policies that reward initiatives for economic change. As elsewhere in China, herdsmen are free to establish their own enterprises if they choose, although financial backing has remained an obstacle. Nonetheless, in 1988 the first trade center for Kazak products run by Kazaks themselves opened in Xinyuan, a town west of Yining, on the Ili River. According to government sources, this was the first center funded and operated by former herdsmen. The men pooled their funds and opened their own trade center to sell everyday items, made to Kazak specifications and taste, and to buy animal products. According to a government report, some 2,000 herdsmen and women had turned into merchants, taking advantage of the new economic freedoms.[32]

In the 1990s, these and other economic activities raised the income of individual herder families. However, as indicated in the following section, the overall income of the Kazaks and other herders has lagged behind that of other groups in Xinjiang. As the government appears to rely on economic change to forestall instability, the continued disparity between herders' and other workers' incomes is a matter of particular concern, both to the government and to the Kazak herders' themselves.

Income

Herders' incomes increased slowly in the reform era. The net per capita income of peasants and herders was 545.61 yuan in 1989.[33] In comparison, in 1987, the average worker in Xinjiang's PCC was earning 1,400 yuan, more than double that of a herder or peasant-farmer.[34] By 1990, Xinjiang's urban workers, the vast majority of whom are Han Chinese, earned 2,007 yuan a year, comparing favorably with the urban per capita income of 1,950 yuan for all of China.[35]

By 1994, net income for the farmers and herdsmen had risen to 936 yuan a year, a substantial increase over the 1989 levels. But the economic reforms had boosted urban income much more rapidly, reaching 4,252 yuan, roughly four times as high as a peasant or herder.[36] This region-wide disparity between rural and urban income is reflected in figures for the Ili-Kazak prefecture. Overall, the income of Ili-Kazak villagers in 1994 was reported as 967 yuan, close to the regional average cited above. While urban income in the prefecture was not as high

Table 5.9

Ili-Kazak Autonomous-Prefecture's Income Levels by District and City, 1994

Area	Income (in Yuan)	Number of Workers (Urban only)
Ili-Kazak prefecture		
Urban	—	468,187
Rural	967	—
Ili district		
Urban	2,293	164,334
Rural	933	—
Tacheng district		
Urban	2,401	120,641
Rural	1,241	—
Altay district		
Urban	—	84,039
Rural	853	—
Kuitun city*	2,969	44,947
Yining city		
Urban	2,293	24,720
Villages	1,157	—
Altay city		
Village	905	16,399
Tacheng city		
Urban	2,403	15,926
Village	1,394	—

Source: *Xinjiang nianjian 1995.*
*Cities include both the city limits and surrounding environs; thus Chinese sources give both "urban" and "rural" figures for cities in the prefecture.

as that of Urumqi, the disparity between rural and urban income was nonetheless pronounced. For instance, in Kuitun, the average income in 1994 was 2,969 yuan. This city of over 90,000 had only 6,362 national minority residents.[37] The incomes by districts and cities within the prefecture reflect similar differences (see table 5.9).

The official figures on income are not the whole story, of course. Interviews in 1996 with Kazaks and Urumqi residents revealed that tax evasion remains a lively pastime. One of the authors was told that Kazak herds had continued to increase, as had prices for mutton and beef, raising incomes for Kazaks living near the regional capital. Taxes, including the slaughter tax, remained very low; nonetheless, some herders avoided even this small tax by illegally slaughtering animals for sale. To combat this, in 1995 all but one slaughterhouse was closed in Urumqi in order to keep better track of animals sold—and of taxes due. Despite such efforts, sheep carcasses are delivered—by motorcycle sidecar and other somewhat incongruous means of transportation—to small butcher shops all over the capital in the early morning hours, in a delivery system that appears extremely difficult to regulate. As in earlier periods of Xinjiang's history, it is also probable that the number of animals in a given herd is not reported accurately, so that the disposable income of some groups of Kazaks may be considerably higher than figures indicate.

Another source of income that may go untaxed is income from the tourist trade. Only Kazaks living at relatively accessible tourist sites can benefit from the increasing numbers of visitors, but renting yurts, horses, and horse-drawn carts can bring in extra cash in the summer months to families who take the initiative to cater to tourists, both domestic and foreign.

Despite the probability of unreported animals and extra income from tourism for some families, the average Kazak income doubtless remains lower than that of the majority Han Chinese and of urban residents in general—as suggested in official figures that consistently report far lower incomes for rural populations. In a 1995 report on the state of the region, over 1 million peasants and herdsmen in Xinjiang were classified as living in poverty.[38] An increasing nationwide gap in earnings between urban and rural populations portends great difficulty for all China; but in Xinjiang, where urban centers remain predominantly Han Chinese, the disparity exacerbates ethnic differences.

Education

Income is linked to education level in China, as elsewhere. Education in urban areas remains generally superior to that available in rural areas. In the 1980s, while efforts have been made by the government to provide education to those Kazaks who continue to follow a nomadic lifestyle or to live in more remote parts of the prefecture, some 20 percent of herders' children received no education at all.

Figures for literacy and education in the Ili-Kazak prefecture prior to 1949 indicate illiteracy rates of up to 80 percent for the Kazaks. According to Chinese sources, the autonomous prefecture had 79 elementary schools in 1944, with a total of 6,200 Kazak students. As a result of efforts by the East Turkestan Republic, by 1949 there were 489 elementary schools, teaching 52,719 students, and 13 middle schools, teaching 1,610 students. Students were of all nationalities except Chinese. Higher education had also taken root in the 1940s: In 1946, Ahmetjan Kasimi had established the Science and Technology Institute at Yining to train specialists in government, education, technology, and animal husbandry. A girls' school was also opened, similar to the one in Urumqi.

After 1949, the numbers of schools and full-time students at all levels in the region continued to grow. However, statistics issued sporadically up to 1980 by the PRC only give the overall number of minority students, making it difficult to trace how many Kazaks were actually receiving an education and at what level.

By 1982, the Ili-Kazak prefecture had 1,571 elementary schools, with 395,645 students of all nationalities; of these schools, 842 were classified as national minority schools, with a Kazak student enrollment of 112,117. The prefecture also had 409 middle schools, with 158,233 students; of these, 204 schools were national minority schools, serving 81,491 students, of whom 38,984 were Kazaks. (Some Kazak students may also attend Han Chinese schools, so these numbers are only approximate). In addition to these city, town, and village schools, the government also set up "tent" schools for Kazaks who continued to follow their herds. By the 1980s, however, the government encouraged Kazak students from nomadic families to attend boarding schools. In 1982, 125 such schools provided education for 29,901 minority students. In the same year, the government reported that 80 percent of herders' children were receiving an education.[39] While the 80 percent figure suggests a degree of success for these efforts, it also meant that one-fifth of herders' children still received no formal education in 1982.

The reasons why not all Kazaks choose to take advantage of educational opportunities are complex. In traditional society, education was prized, and those who had religious or other formal training were highly regarded. Resistance to formal training was not an issue; rather, the opportunities were so limited that few families could provide their children with education. After 1949, as more schools were built and elementary education was popularized, Kazaks began attending school in larger numbers, as indicated by the figures above. However, attending school also meant studying the Chinese language, required for all minority students, and a considerable amount of political indoctrination. Elementary school texts from the 1960s and 1970s for Kazak children included stories about Chairman Mao and the party and were filled with implicit admiration of and devotion to the communist cause. For Kazaks, for whom Muslim faith is a matter of self and cultural identity, the atheist message of communism was unacceptable. Also, receiving an education meant the separation of children from their families for at least part of the year. The loss of sons' and daughters' labor, plus the inevitable indoctrination of the curriculum, made the promise of a better life through education an empty one for many families.

For Kazaks who did choose to send their children to school, another challenge was to find a school in which the pupils were educated in their own language, at least at the elementary level. There was a severe shortage of trained minority teachers; and, despite government efforts, minority teacher education remained a problem. As late as 1982, out of 31,547 teachers in the autonomous prefecture, only 10,124 were Kazak. To increase the number of minority teachers, the Ili area established a two-year institute of education for training middle-school teachers.

Although there has been some resistance to state schools, for reasons indicated above, education levels among the Kazaks appear to be rising, as has the availability of education beyond the primary level. The prefecture has established a number of technical schools, providing training in electronics, mechanics, telecommunications, and so on. The total number of students enrolled in the latter schools in the early 1980s was 1,667; by 1983 there were 3,750 minority graduates from these technical programs.

The highest level of education offered in the Ili-Kazak prefecture is at the Ili Teachers' Training College, which, in 1980, had 908 students who were taught in the Kazak, Han (Chinese), and Uyghur languages. This has remained the highest level of locally available education, so students wishing to pursue further study must go to Urumqi or to other universities in China. In 1978, the government announced that national minorities could use their own language to take the university entrance exam and that they would be given preferential treatment.[40] Although in the 1990s, minority students can enter university with lower scores than their Han Chinese counterparts, they must often spend an initial year at university studying Chinese so that they will be able to read and take examinations at the same level of Chinese-language competence as Han students.[41]

A small number of Kazaks have pursued education beyond the bachelor's degree, but no statistics are yet available. In the 1990s, Dr. Baket was the first Kazak to receive a Ph.D. degree in the region, beginning a new era for Kazak intellectual leadership. As noted earlier, other Kazaks are taking advantage of opportunities to study in the universities of neighboring Kazakstan.

Overall, increasing levels of education will enable Kazaks to take advantage of the changes now occurring in Xinjiang—advancing themselves in trade and business and providing leadership for the Kazak areas, and perhaps even influencing the course of changes that will affect Kazak culture. As important as education is, however, the key to Kazaks' role in the prefecture will be their decision either to participate in or to oppose their local government and the CCP. The Kazaks' collective future in China may depend on the ability of the next generation of young Kazak leaders to assert their own agendas through local institutions and, especially, local government, a topic to which we now turn.

Ili-Kazak Prefectural Government and Party

Participation of minorities in political and governmental institutions is one measure of their integration into—or acceptance of—the greater social system. As noted earlier, over the years the CCP has cultivated members of every minority for positions in the party, government, and military. By 1982, the total number of national minority party members in the prefecture was 30,636, of which 18,171 were Kazaks.[42] In addition to minority party membership, the number of minority cadre provides another measure of minority participation in the present system. According to the official history of the Ili-Kazak Autonomous Prefecture published in 1985, the area had 10,926 national minority cadres before the prefecture was established; no breakdown by ethnic group was given. By 1982, however, the number of minority cadre was 39,469, or 50.6 percent of the prefectural total; of these, 21,796 were Kazaks, or 55.3 percent. Of the Kazak cadre, 1,679 were classified as "leading cadre" or as officials with higher-level positions of responsibility in the prefectural government.[43]

In 1988, the secretary of the party committee in Ili was a Han Chinese, Wu Guihe.[44] In 1995, possibly because the dissolution of the USSR brought new geopolitical realities to the Ili region, a native of the region, Kankejan (Kangkejian), was named secretary of the Ili-Kazak party committee. Another Kazak, Beg Mehmet Musa (Biekemuhamaiti musa), had become chair of the prefectural government in 1994.[45] The Tacheng district deputy secretary was also of minority nationality—Rabat Bay Rahim (Lebusibailahemu). Overall, by 1995 there were 269,000 minority cadre in the region, or 46.8 percent of the total.[46]

The PLA and PCC in the Ili-Kazak
Autonomous Prefecture

Within the prefecture's borders are farms and ranches belonging to four of the ten divisions of the Xinjiang PCC. In 1949, the military established its initial four farms in Xinjiang. The GMD troops stranded in Xinjiang in September 1949, when their leaders chose to go over to the CCP, provided the basic labor force for these enterprises, in which thousands of men began the arduous, back-breaking work of reclaiming land, building roads across deserts, and working on irrigation projects in some of the most inhospitable terrain in China. In recognition of his decision to support the CCP, the former GMD commander in Xinjiang, Tao Zhiyue, was made commander of this paramilitary force.

In 1954 the PCC was officially established under its new name, the Production Construction Corps of the People's Liberation Army. The 200,000 men of the corps were divided into ten divisions: Five were from the First Field Army Corps of the PLA; four were former GMD troops; and one was composed of minority nationalities. The men were to spend three-fourths of their time on farming and reconstruction work and one-fourth on military training.[47]

There are PCC farms in all three districts of the prefecture, as shown in maps from the 1980s. In Altay, there are military farms 181 and 182; in Tacheng, along the former Soviet border, are farms 166 and 168, while further away from the border are farms 124, 126, 133, and 170; in Ili, there are two farms near the former Soviet border, numbers 63 and 74.[48] The ethnic composition of these units is known in a few instances; in general, minority participation in these largely

Han enterprises has remained limited. The Fourth Division, based at Yining, had a total of 212,440 members in 1989. Of these, 14 percent (29,741) are listed as belonging to minority nationalities, but no breakdown by ethnic group is given.[49] The only other PCC division for which we have figures on Kazak members is the small Tenth Agricultural Division based in the city of Altay, capital of the Altay district. In this unit, .09 percent are said to be Kazak, a total of only sixty people.[50] Another unit mentioning Kazaks specifically is the Seventh Agricultural Division, based at Kuitun, the city directly under the prefectural administration. This division had a total of 193,688 members in 1989, of which minorities were 3.55 percent or 6,876 people.[51] Kazak participation in the PCC appears to be greatest in areas outside the Kazak autonomous units. For instance, in the Fifth Division, based in the Bortala-Mongol Autonomous Prefecture (which is bordered on all sides by the Ili-Kazak prefecture), there were 69,443 members in 1989, of which 3.7 percent were Kazak, a total of 2,569 people.[52]

Higher pay is doubtless the main reason why Kazaks join the PCC. The average income in these units in 1989 was 843 yuan, but at Bortala and Altay the average was over 1,000.[53] Compared to the average for peasants and herders in the same year (545 yuan), the advantages in terms of income are clear.

The exact percentage of the PCC's overall economic contribution to the Ili-Kazak prefecture is unclear. Region-wide, the PCC's impact is enormous: By 1990, approximately 18 percent of the region's population were employed by the PCC, and its output accounted for up to one-fourth of the region's agricultural and industrial output, by value.[54] Although the specific contribution of the PCC units within the prefecture is not available, the fact that ten PCC units are now well established there suggests that the corps' impact is considerable.

What also remains unclear about the PCC is how minorities join. Some may be descendants of former East Turkestani military, rewarded by the government in memory of these early revolutionaries; others may come from those families whose sympathies toward the CCP were declared early. Available sources do not make clear the means by which a minority nationality may join lucrative PCC operations in their area. As reported in earlier chapters, opposition to the PCC has been voiced consistently within the Xinjiang-Uyghur region, and the increasing disparity in income between PCC and private family herds may contribute to ongoing Kazak opposition to a PCC presence.

Ethnonationalism in the Ili-Kazak
Autonomous Prefecture

As noted earlier, the CCP has attached special importance to the Ili area, in part because of the legacy of the East Turkestani movement based there in the 1940s. In the increasingly open atmosphere of the reform era, the government has had to remain vigilant. Constantly it has reiterated its official interpretation of the events of 1944–1949, stressing the party-sanctioned views of past Muslim leaders in an effort to maintain control over both the past and the present in the Ili area.

From the beginning, all official discussion of the East Turkestan Republic was couched in revolutionary rhetoric, co-opting it as part of the Chinese people's revolution in 1949. But at the same time, detailed accounts of the movement were suppressed. For decades, publications mentioning the East Turkestan Republic referred to it only as the Three Districts Revolution and gave only the briefest CCP-approved interpretation of events. Decades after the events themselves—and after most of the leaders had passed away—discussion of the republic broadened. By the 1980s, more information was available than ever before. Initially this was through the officially sanctioned publication of local histories, which included brief accounts of key events. In 1986, the regional museum in Urumqi held an exhibition on the Three Districts Revolution, displaying weapons, personal effects of leaders like Ahmetjan Kasimi, and a wealth of photographs. In 1994, on the fiftieth anniversary of the founding of the East Turkestan Republic, the Xinjiang-Uyghur Autonomous Region issued *Xinjiang sanqu geming dashiji* (Great events in the Xinjiang Three Districts Revolution) and an illustrated volume entitled *Xinjiang sanqu geming* (Xinjiang's Three Districts Revolution), both in Chinese and Uyghur. These books, along with an increasing number of articles in academic journals on this once-forbidden and restricted topic, attest to the passing away of the generation who were witness to the events; but they are also an indication of the continued power of the memory of the East Turkestan Republic and its leaders. The more open atmosphere of the reform era has meant constant vigilance on the part of the government in an effort to combat increasing ethnonationalism among the various groups that participated, including the Kazaks.

Since the early 1980s, Kazaks have participated in demonstrations leading in some instances to violent confrontations with Han Chinese civilians and officials. An account of some of these incidents is given in chapter 6, which suggests that as the Kazak areas continue to change, the government will need to pay more attention to the issues that most deeply affect the Kazaks.

Conclusion

The Ili-Kazak Autonomous Prefecture is an area of huge economic potential, which is now being realized in part through the efforts of the PCC, government encouragement of local enterprises, cross-border trade (see chapter 7), and improved infrastructure. The policy in the 1990s of relying on continued economic development and expansion to foster better relations between Kazak and Han Chinese, however, could also have the opposite effect, exaggerating differences in access to power brokers and capital that favor Han and highlighting the growing disparity in income between rural and urban populations.

Above all, the system of autonomy that ostensibly guaranteed Kazaks a role in the development and administration of the prefecture is now redundant. Despite the fact that the prefecture remains the single most important Kazak area in China, the greatly increased Han Chinese presence makes the Kazaks a minority. The 1990s have seen no diminuation in the numbers of Han, who in 1991 numbered 1.49 million—far outnumbering the 896,140 Kazaks.[55] In 1994, the Han population was 1.57 million (44 percent of the total), an increase of 5 percent in just three years. Kazak population figures for the same year indicate a total of 934,000 (26 percent of the total). However, as noted earlier, the figures for the Han Chinese population exclude predominantly Han groups such as the PLA military units, the members of PCC farms and ranches, and the involuntary residents of the laogai camps and prisons. More than any other factor, this dramatic change in the ethnic composition of the prefecture colors every aspect of economic and political development there.

The Barkol-Kazak Autonomous County

The Barkol-Kazak Autonomous County (Balikun-Hasake zizhixian), which is separated from the Ili-Kazak Autonomous Prefecture by some 900 kilometers, is part of the Hami district, the easternmost district of Xinjiang. It was established in the same year as the Ili prefecture, on

September 30, 1954. Like the Ili prefecture, the Hami district also has an international border: a 605-kilometer stretch shared with Mongolia along its northern edge. To the east, the district borders the neighboring province of Gansu, with which it shares a vast stretch of the Gobi Desert. The district capital, known locally as Komul but called Hami by the Chinese authorities, has a long history as an oasis on the ancient trade route linking China to Central Asia and the Middle East. In 1990, its population of approximately 300,000 was composed of 66 percent Han, 26 percent Uyghur, and 2.7 percent Kazak, as well as 5.3 percent of eight other nationalities. In 1994, the city's population had grown to 314,334, of which 103,779 people belonged to minority nationalities.[56]

The Barkol-Kazak Autonomous County lies to the north of Hami, covering 38,440 square kilometers. The southern border of the county is just to the north of the region's major east-west highway and railroad, both of which arteries angle slightly north, eventually following along the southwestern edge of the county's border. In the north the county borders Mongolia. In 1991, the county's population was 103,982, including over 73,000 Han and nearly 28,000 Kazaks. Figures for 1994 indicate a drop in population, to 100,446, of which 29,846 were classified as minorities, with no ethnic group breakdown provided.[57]

Topographically, the county is divided roughly into thirds: desert and rocky wasteland in the north; mountains and mountain pastures in the south; and flatlands and marshy areas, much of the latter surrounding Barkol Lake, in the south-central area.[58] The lake's environs have long been desirable for grazing, providing some 20,000 mu of pasture, some of it mixed with swamplands. The lake area is also a source of Glauber's salt (mirabilite). One hundred thirty square kilometers are covered with the mineral, which is processed and sold by the Hami Chemical Works.[59]

The county's capital is the town of Barkol, which, like the district capital of Hami, was also a stop on the ancient Silk Road. The town is both the administrative and economic center.

Kazaks first moved into the Barkol area in the nineteenth century. At that time, Barkol and Hami were both under the control of Uyghur hereditary nobility, in the person of the prince of Hami, whose title and right to tax the inhabitants of Barkol was conferred by the Qing dynasty. During the rebellion of Yakub Beg in the 1870s, the Qing general Zuo Zongtang used Barkol as a staging post, transporting grain to both Barkol and Qitai to supply his men during the campaign to reassert Chinese control in Xinjiang.[60]

In the twentieth century, Barkol was once more drawn into a Chinese-Muslim confrontation when the Chinese governor, Jin Shuren, attempted to remove the prince of Hami from power. In 1931 this resulted in widespread revolt against the Han provincial authorities, who managed to quell the rebellion only after great bloodshed. Hami was heavily damaged in the fighting, as was the village of Barkol and the surrounding area. After the fighting ended, Kazaks once more grazed flocks near Barkol Lake. In the 1940s, the Kazak leader Osman Batur moved into the Barkol area, using it as a base for his operations against the East Turkestan Republic in 1947.

Although the area has been used by Kazaks off and on since the nineteenth century, the number of Kazaks in Barkol county was never very large. The pre-1949 population of Han Chinese at Barkol was already over 10,000, while Kazaks numbered less than 5,000. Nonetheless, after 1949, Barkol was designated a Kazak autonomous county, a status that continued despite an overwhelmingly Han Chinese population (see table 5.10).

As in other autonomous areas, efforts were made by the new government at an early stage to include minorities in the party and civil government. Thus when Barkol's people elected their county-level people's congress in 1954, ten of the nineteen members were Kazaks. Their 52 percent share of the total seats was far greater than their proportion in the county population, which was then only about 31 percent. The chairman of the county was also Kazak, seconded as in all such situations, by a Han Chinese deputy.

Unlike the Ili area, however, which had experienced a locally led, locally run government, the Barkol area had been Chinese dominated prior to 1949. With no trained individuals to rely upon for assistance in the transformation of the county, the CCP turned for leadership to members of the landlord class—or to be more precise, the herd-owner class. One of the earliest such individuals called upon was Hawan, a Kazak who was instrumental in easing the way for the CCP in the county from 1949 onwards. Born in 1925, Hawan was from Mori, another Kazak area (discussed below as the Mori-Kazak Autonomous County). In the old society he had been a landlord and herd-owner; one Chinese source adds that he had even beaten his seasonal laborers and oppressed the people.[61] He "changed completely" after 1949 and

Table 5.10

Barkol-Kazak Autonomous County Population

Ethnic Group	1944	1982	1991	1994
Han	11,695	60,900	73,127	70,600
Kazak	4,941	20,100	27,878	—
Uyghur	283	303	1,302	—
Hui	—	492	355	—
Mongol	78	790	1,250	—
Tatar	—	90	—	—
Manchu	—	—	19	—
Other	—	—	51	29,846*
Total	16,961	91,000	103,982	100,446

Sources: Figures for 1944 are from *Tianshan yuegan* (October 15, 1947), 10–13. The 1982 figures are from *Balikun-Hasake zizhixian* (1984), 108. The 1991 figures are from *Xinjiang nianjian* (1992), 40. The 1994 figures are from *Xinjian nianjian* (1995), p. 451.

*No ethnic breakdown is provided for 1994, other than Han and all other nationalities; numbers are as in the original sources and do not always add up to the final figure given in the source.

began to work for the party. Under CCP guidance, he worked to persuade a group of forty Kazak households in Sujizaoyuan to establish the county's first mutual-aid team and went on to establish an animal husbandry cooperative. He was accepted into the party in 1955. He then served in various capacities in the Barkol county government, including stints as deputy county head, county party committee secretary, vice-chairman of the county assembly, member of the county Nationality Affairs Commission, and representative to the National People's Congress. He remained active in county affairs until his death in 1979.

Stories like that of Hawan are informative. Clearly the CCP had to rely on those Kazaks willing to cooperate with the party's new agenda, regardless of class background. While the fact that Hawan led households to join the mutual-aid team movement was no doubt useful for the CCP, his change of allegiance appears to have taken place only after Kazak resistance had been eliminated in the area and the necessity of compromise with the new government was clear.

Kazaks, however, played a less important role overall than did the military, which in 1950–1951 moved into villages throughout the county in order to "investigate conditions and carry out land reform." The subsequent "good works" of the military stationed in Barkol were featured in media reports. The reality was less prosaic: The military presence was necessary to ensure control over the Kazak and Uyghur populations, preventing them from joining or in any way supporting Muslim groups opposed to the new government.

Following the precedence established elsewhere in Xinjiang, Barkol's population was urged to organize into mutual-aid teams for herders, the first of which was organized in 1952. By 1955, there were twenty-one, one-third of which formed only in that same year. The twenty-one teams reportedly accounted for 95 percent of all Barkol herder families. Subsequently, many Barkol herding families joined cooperatives, so that by 1957, 1,121 households (92 percent) were in some form of cooperative. The pace of reform was faster than in the Ili area and appears to have been carried out with relatively little resistance on the part of local herding families, who were, after all, far outnumbered in the county by other nationalities.

The goal of these new economic units was to increase the herds of the members, and initially this appears to have been the case: The total number of animals in the county rose from 151,000 animals before 1949 to 215,000 in 1954 and 381,000 in 1958. However, the Great Leap Forward had a huge negative impact on the area, and the number of animals fell to 188,000 in 1965. By the end of the 1970s, herds had recovered, with a total animal population of 488,000 by 1979.[62] The numbers here reflect the political fortunes of the region as it suffered first under the Great Leap and then under the Cultural Revolution.

Barkol was also affected in other ways by the Cultural Revolution, as local political elites were drawn into the struggle. Although the number of minorities who suffered as a result is not available, a total of 1,410 cases of "errors" against cadre in Barkol were discovered after the Cultural Revolution ended. Most likely, the majority of these victims were Han Chinese, as was the case elsewhere in the autonomous region. Nonetheless, the impact was great enough in the Barkol area that efforts by the CCP to repair damage to the economy—and to the CCP's reputation—continued well into the 1980s. Chinese media reports stressed the respect with which all national minority customs and habits were treated, and efforts to recruit Kazak cadre and CCP members began anew. Barkol's recovery was faster than in Ili; and by the end of the 1970s, the county was developing rapidly, fostering a small but growing manufacturing base and an expanding agricultural sector as a basis for even faster economic growth in the era of reform.

Barkol in the Reform Era

Beginning in the 1980s, Barkol county began economic expansion that relied primarily on light industry and agriculture, rather than on animal husbandry. As a result of government efforts, Barkol's animal- and animal-product-based economy was diversified, with the county now producing coal, charcoal, cement, cotton cloth, and various processed foods—150 products altogether. Output was valued at over 7 million yuan in 1979, fifteen times the output of 1949. By 1994, the output was valued at 1.5 billion. The number of minorities engaged in these new lines of production is not available; but given the preponderance of Han Chinese in the county, it seems likely that Han Chinese predominate in the new areas of employment.

The PCC has also played a role in the county's development, but the extent of its role is unclear. No PCC farms are shown on recent maps of the county; on the other hand, a recent yearbook notes that birth and death rates for the county exclude the population of the PCC border divisions—units that are not mentioned anywhere else in the entry for Barkol.[63] Possibly the PCC in Barkol remains more military than industrial or agricultural, playing an increasingly vital role as Mongolia continues to accelerate its democratization and development outside of the communist orbit.

Formal education has also made progress in Barkol, but the amount of education received by minorities is unclear. From a low of only 45 elementary students and 90 middle-school students in 1949, the total number of students in elementary school rose to 460 by 1952, and middle-school students numbered over 290. By 1965, there were 27 elementary schools, with over 7,000 students; of these, seven schools were for Kazaks only, with a combined enrollment of 1,500 students. Middle-school education lagged behind, with only 110 Kazaks in middle school in the same year. After the Cultural Revolution, enrollments among Kazaks increased, so that there were 3,379 Kazak elementary students enrolled in 1979; 549 Kazaks were attending the middle schools. Altogether, the government asserted that 92 percent of Barkol's Kazak school-age children were in school and that 82 percent of its Kazak population had an elementary education.[64]

Barkol Kazak Participation in the Party and Government

In 1950, the total number of CCP cadre in Barkol was 113, a number that included all nationalities. Over the next few decades, care was taken to cultivate an appropriate number of minority cadre. By 1979, the government reported that of 1,691 cadre, 363 were from various national minorities, accounting for 20 percent of all cadres in the county. Given both the lack of figures on minority cadre and the now-overwhelming Han Chinese presence in Barkol, it seems likely that the Kazaks are only a marginal economic and political presence in Barkol today. Incomes have risen overall in the county in the era of reform, as have opportunities for making money and acquiring an education. At the same time, no incidents of ethnic violence or even demonstrations have appeared in the media for Barkol, indicating Kazaks' contentment with—of at least their acceptance of—the current conditions in the county.

Conclusion

Unlike the Ili area, there is little to indicate that Kazaks in Barkol are discontent with Chinese policies in the way Ili Kazaks have been. Too few in number to be able to organize effectively, the Kazaks here have relied on the guarantee of political participation ensured by the autonomy system as a means to influence events or, more often, to improve their own personal situation. The improved living standards since 1978, the fact that the Han were already a majority in the county prior to 1949, and the relative isolation of Barkol appear to be the most important factors contributing to its relative stability in an era of rapid change for the Xinjiang-Uyghur Autonomous Region.

Mori-Kazak Autonomous County

The Mori-Kazak Autonomous County (Mulei-Hasake zizhixian) was established on June 17, 1954, the first of the Kazak autonomous units established in Xinjiang. Just as the Barkol-Kazak Autonomous County is under the jurisdiction of the Hami district, the Mori-Kazak Autonomous County is a subdivision of the Changji-Hui Autonomous Prefecture—a 77,500-square-kilometer area that is sandwiched between the Hami prefecture to the east and the Ili-Kazak prefecture to the west. The Changji-Hui prefecture's southern border abuts the city limits of Urumqi, which is not under Changji jurisdiction but is a self-contained political unit. Like the Hami district, the Changji-Hui prefecture also shares part of the Mongolian border along its northernmost edge. In 1994 the prefecture had a total population of 1.36 million.[65] The prefectural capital of Changji has a population of some 200,000 people. Like other newly urban areas, its population is overwhelmingly Han and mirrors the ethnic composition of the prefecture: In 1989 the city was 76 percent Han, 14 percent Hui, 6 percent Kazak, 3 percent Uyghur, and contained a number of other nationalities.[66]

Mori-Kazak Autonomous County, one of eight counties in the prefecture, is the only one designated as autonomous. Covering 33,613 square kilometers, its 1994 population was 87,865, of which 25,709 were minority nationalities.[67] Its capital is the town of Mori, located at the far eastern end of the prefecture. On the other side of the county's border is neighboring Hami district's Barkol-Kazak Autonomous County, which is connected to Mori by two secondary roads but not by a main highway. Except for political purposes, it is unclear why these two were not joined to make a separate Kazak prefecture.

In addition to the Mori-Kazak county, the prefecture also has eight townships designated as Kazak autonomous units. These are scattered from east to west, mainly in the Tian Shan and its foothills, where Kazak herds pasture.[68] Kazaks also live in many other areas of the prefecture that are outside the Mori-Kazak county and the autonomous Kazak townships. The tourist site of Tianchi Lake, for example, provides Kazaks with summer pastures and the opportunity to make extra money by catering to visitors. The valley of Miao'er, southeast of Changji city, is another area where Kazak herds graze on the northern slopes of the Tian Shan.

The PRC depiction of life for Kazaks in the Mori area prior to the arrival of the CCP in 1949 is grim. According to an official account published in 1984, less than 10 percent of the Kazaks owned 90 percent of the area herds. The vast majority lived in thrall to the great herd owners, who expected both payment of taxes in kind as well as labor. For farmers, the situation appears to have been much better, with 95 percent of the peasants holding 75 percent of the land (which still left 4.5 percent of the population to control 23 percent of the land, the same source pointed out).[69]

After liberation in 1949, the area received its first group of CCP cadre; by March 1950 the first "all county, all nationality, all circles" people's representative assembly was held to select a temporary people's government committee and to establish lower level governments throughout the county. However, in April of that year, as spring plowing was about to commence, Osman and Yolbars Khan, allies of the defeated Guomindang, brought chaos to Mori. According to the county's 1984 official history, the local population appealed to the government to eliminate these bandits. Therefore, in May 1950, the PLA arrived in Mori and, joined by members of the local people's militia, began the hunt for Osman. The military operation was called the Military Suppression and United Political Thought Movement, relying on the "suppress while uniting" method. This was explained as simultaneously using military suppression and organizing committees of Kazaks and herd owners to suppress the bandits themselves. The official accounts make it difficult to judge the actual levels of participation and support for such activities among the Kazaks during this early period. It is clear, however, that bandit suppression continued well after Osman had been captured and executed and Yolbars had fled the country. The military campaign continued into the spring of 1953, indicating that other groups besides the two infamous "bandits" were also waging a minor war of resistance. The Han troops based at Qitai, a town near Mori, had heavy enough losses to produce a number of martyrs to the revolution. Out of twenty-nine martyrs who died near Mori and Hami (which includes the Barkol-Kazak area) in the early 1950s, twenty-three were Chinese. Only one Kazak, a man named Sunya Ahmet, who died in Qitai county, is listed as a revolutionary martyr, suggesting limited participation in this phase of the bandit suppression campaign in Mori.[70]

The county's farming population was relatively small in 1949–1950, and it is therefore likely that, as reported by the government, land reform was quickly accomplished. After the first year, the landowners' 302,760 hectares had been redistributed to 976 households. Likewise, 221 plowing animals, over 3,000 pieces of farm equipment, and 272,540 jin of food were all divided among 1,836 farm households.[71]

Work also began immediately to train Kazak cadre to work with those herders who remained outside the farming community. Only eleven minority cadre were identified in the area in 1950, and work to recruit members from among the county's Kazaks did not apparently make much headway. By the 1980s, there were still only 308 minority cadre, and only 29.9 percent of these were party members. The Cultural Revolution was particularly violent in the county, and this was doubtless one of the reasons why the CCP recruitment efforts continued to have only limited success.

By 1954, enough progress had been made to allow for the establishment of local people's government in the Mori area. At the county's first consultative people's assembly in 1954, there were eighty-one people's representatives. Kazaks accounted for 34 percent of the population, but they were nonetheless allotted 48.9 percent of the seats; Han, 55 percent of the population, held 38.6 percent of the seats. When twenty-one people were chosen at the first meeting in July 1954 to lead the county, the group included a Kazak chairman, Rajip (Rejiafu), as well as eleven other Kazaks, six Han, two Uyghur, and one Uzbek. The need to follow official guidelines, which required that the autonomous county government be led by Kazaks, predominated over the reality of the area's actual ethnic composition.

As in the other Kazak areas of Xinjiang, the same general policies of economic reorganization were carried out in the Mori-Kazak county. Mori's total population was smaller than that of Barkol, with only 22,000 residents in 1953. Of these, less than 7,100 were Kazak. Thus, work to organize mutual-aid teams went faster than in the sensitive Ili districts. Initially, twelve households of herders were organized into two mutual-aid teams, and each of these was given 250 sheep. Three more teams were quickly organized after this. Another 304 herder households were given loans to establish themselves in agriculture. By 1955, there were thirty-six mutual-aid teams, which both farmed and raised animals. By 1956, the number of mutual-aid teams had risen to forty-seven, representing 375 families. The success of the teams up to that point resulted in 75 percent of the county's Kazaks joining co-ops that same year. By 1958, twenty-four pastoral communes were organized, incorporating 86 percent of the herders. That same year the Bostan (Bositang) Company, a joint state-private enterprise, attracted eighteen herd owners, who together contributed a total of 18,500 animals as the company's capital.[72]

As elsewhere in Xinjiang, the number of Han Chinese throughout the Changji prefecture increased in the late 1950s. Towns and villages all along the main east-west road experienced considerable growth. In the western part of the prefecture, cities like Changji and Manas grew quickly; smaller towns in the east of the prefecture like Qitai and Jimsar also saw increases in their populations, aided by improved roads linking these areas to the regional capital of Urumqi.

This pattern extended to Mori as well. By 1979 there were over 57,000 Han Chinese residents, a dramatic increase over the less than

Table 5.11

Mori-Kazak Autonomous County Population Growth by Ethnic Group, 1944–1991

Nationality	1944	1953	1982	1991
Kazaks	4,109	7,055	12,975	18,494
Han	4,958	11,582	57,210	62,826
Uyghur	1,483	1,853	3,626	4,082
Hui	40	—	—	790
Mongol	199	—	—	9
Uzbek	—	—	—	1,073
Tatar	—	—	—	75
Manchu	—	—	—	26
Other	13	568	1,050	151
Total	10,802	21,058	74,861	87,526

Sources: The 1944 figures are from *Tianshan yuekan* (Tianshan monthly) 1 (October 15, 1947): 10–13. The 1953 figures are from I.B. Shevel, "Nacional'noe stroitel'stvo v Sin'czjanskom Ujgurskom Avtonomnom Rajone Kitajskoj Narodnoj Respubliki" (National construction in the Xinjiang-Uyghur Autonomous Region of the People's Republic of China), *Sovetskaja etnografija* (Soviet ethnography) 2 (1956): 99. The 1982 figures are from *Mulei Hasake zizhixian gaikuang* (A survey of Mori-Kazak Autonomous County) (Urumqi: 1984), 2. The 1991 figures are from *Xinjiang nianjian 1992* (Xinjiang yearbook for 1992), 40–41.

5,000 living there in the 1940s. The Kazak population increased as well, but in 1979 there were still only 13,000 Kazaks in the county, a drastic change from the nearly fifty-fifty balance of Han and Kazak in the 1940s (see table 5.11).

Many of the Han settlers in the Changji-Hui prefecture joined the PCC, working on farms and ranches as part of Xinjiang's increasing paramilitary force. As of 1985 none of these enterprises appeared to be based within the Mori-Kazak area, but maps reveal numerous PCC farms elsewhere in the prefecture. West of the prefectural capital were farms number 102, 222, 103, and 105; just to the east, were farms 111, 106, 148, 149, and 150. Near Qitai were farms 108, 110, and 109—the latter only forty-four kilometers from Mori city.[73] Han Chinese also went to work in the area's mines. Among other ores, the county has deposits of iron, coal, copper, lime, salt, gypsum, gold, and silver. The North Mountain coal mine produced over 2 million tons of coal by the 1970s, and the Great Stone commune mined ten different kinds of ore.

Cultural Revolution and Reform Era Changes in Mori-Kazak Autonomous County

Mori-Kazak county's location near the regional capital was doubtless a factor in its being deeply affected by the Cultural Revolution. Its overwhelming Han population, much of it from coastal cities, also meant that the political conflict took a greater toll in terms of production than in Kazak areas with fewer Han. The greatest losses in terms of what had been an increasing agricultural production occurred between 1966 and 1974. In 1966, the county produced a total of 54 million jin of food products, but in 1974 this had fallen to 19 million jin.[74] Clearly, the Han Chinese population was drawn into the political turmoil that accompanied this period, drastically reducing the grain production.

The number of Kazaks who became embroiled in the political struggle is not known, but local Kazaks and their herds were both affected, with huge losses recorded for these years. Mori's animal population had reached a high of 350,000 in 1933, falling to 198,000 in 1944 and dropping to only 65,000 by 1949. As in other Kazak areas, the number of animals reflected periods of turmoil. After 1949, herds began to recover, reaching 116,800 animals by 1953 and over 300,000 by 1965. Losses in the Cultural Revolution were so heavy that ten years after the revolution officially ended in Xinjiang, herds had still not returned to 1965 levels; the 1979 count was only 280,000.[75] In contrast, agricultural production fully recovered, reaching a record of over 92 million jin in 1979.[76]

Likewise, commune income also began to rise after the resolution of the Cultural Revolution. From 1977 to 1980, total income for one of the county's communes rose from 713,721 to 929,754 yuan. Average income for commune members rose from 81 yuan in 1977 to 118 yuan in 1980.

The reform era brought further economic changes to the county. In 1979, the government announced that the old commune system was to be modified in Mori. Exactly when this was done is unclear, but among the first steps taken was lowering of state purchase quotas and granting greater self-determination for peasants to decide what crops to plant. The improved levels of income that resulted led to the purchase of more vehicles in the county, so that by 1984 the county agriculturalists could boast a total of 14 cars, 342 tractors, and numerous other smaller mechanized vehicles.[77]

Education

Chinese sources contend that 95 percent of Mori county's population was illiterate in 1949, a figure that is difficult to prove or dispute because of shortage of data. Prior to 1949, the county reportedly had eleven schools and twenty-four teachers, three of whom were of minority nationalities. These schools served over 600 students, of which 31 were Kazak. By 1956, the number in elementary school had doubled, and some students were continuing on to middle school. In 1956, 141 were enrolled at that level, one-third of whom were Kazak. By the 1960s, there were twenty-nine elementary schools serving 4,500 students.

For the period through the Cultural Revolution there is little information on education at any level. But with the end of the violence and a return to a more rational and, for minorities, a more reconciliatory policy, the region could report in 1981 that it administered seventeen elementary schools in pastoral areas and forty-one in urban and agricultural areas, serving a total of 20,305 students. Among these were 4,315 minority members. The county had established three middle schools for only national minority students; two middle-schools with mixed student populations of Han and minorities; and eleven middle schools for only Han students. Elementary teachers numbered 1,396, of whom 205 were from various minority nationalities. There was a total of 120 middle-school teachers. Although the practice of providing official statistics that place all minorities together in a single category makes it difficult to assess fully the extent or quality of education for the Kazaks in this autonomous county, it appears that progress has been made in educating Mori's Kazak population.

Conclusion

Overall, Mori county has undergone tremendous change since 1949. Its transformation from an isolated herding area into an agricultural and industrial center producing thousands of pounds of foodstuffs and tons of ore to fuel Xinjiang's gradual emergence as an industrial and manufacturing center has been accomplished primarily by Han Chinese settlers whose success can be expected to draw continuing numbers of Chinese to the area. For Kazaks living in the county, continued adaptation to Mori's ongoing metamorphosis will be vital to their maintaining a voice for themselves in what has become a predominantly Han environment.

**The Three Autonomous Kazak Areas—
Concluding Remarks**

In attempting to assess significant differences in the experiences of the Kazaks in Xinjiang's three autonomous Kazak areas since 1949, this chapter has indicated that the histories of each area played a role in setting the stage for CCP-Kazak interaction. In the Ili area, the CCP took into account the area's recent experience as an independent state and initially moved with caution. As a result, the area was slower to reorganize as a socialist economy than the two other Kazak areas. By the 1960s, however, all three units had made the transition.

All the Kazak areas experienced the excesses of Chinese political movements, beginning in the 1950s and continuing into the 1970s. Again, the Ili area's more sensitive past appears to have played a role, reinforced—from a Chinese perspective—by the attempt in 1962 of many Kazaks and Uyghurs to leave and join family and friends across the border in the Kazak Soviet Socialist Republic. Distance from the border precluded this as an option for Kazaks in other areas of Xinjiang, who may have suffered more in the Cultural Revolution than Kazaks in Ili, partly because they lived in predominantly Han areas. In general, up to 1978, CCP policy required conformity with national policies and the government's socialist agenda, but the degree of enforcement varied in Kazak areas depending on particular circumstances.

In all three Kazak areas, the new Han settlers play an important economic role. In developing new industry and mining and in expanding agricultural land and output, the government has relied on Han labor, and this has already transformed the three local economies. Significantly, while the government has sought to include minorities in all its economic experiments, only in the reform era have Kazaks shown much enthusiasm for government-dictated change. Kazaks are embracing the idea of "getting rich" in ways that indicate an eagerness not only to return to the days of privately held herds, but also to establish their own organizations to handle trade and to use their own contacts to do business in Kazakstan.

Although conditions in the Kazak areas have improved greatly under Dengist policies, better economic conditions and higher incomes have not made Chinese attempts to control and shape Kazak cultural expression any more welcome than in previous times. While few reports of unrest have surfaced from the Mori and Barkol areas—both of which have only small numbers of Kazaks relative to the Han and other nationalities—the 1980s and 1990s have seen an escalation of incidents in the Ili area. Much of this unrest revolves around aspects of Kazak culture that the Chinese authorities have sought to control or eliminate, as discussed in more detail in chapter 6. The death of Deng in early 1997 is unlikely to bring a change in Chinese policy toward the Kazaks or other minorities in China. Although international media are including more coverage of minority issues in China—particularly on Tibet, but increasingly on the northwest and other regions, as well as on the new republics of Central Eurasia—the past experience of the Kazaks gives little reason to expect any change in the Chinese approach to minority issues in Xinjiang.

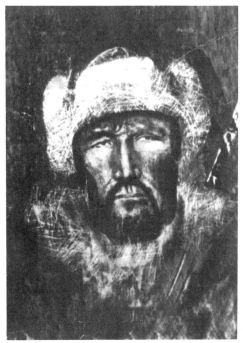

Osman Batur. Black and white photo of a sketch of the Kazak leader.

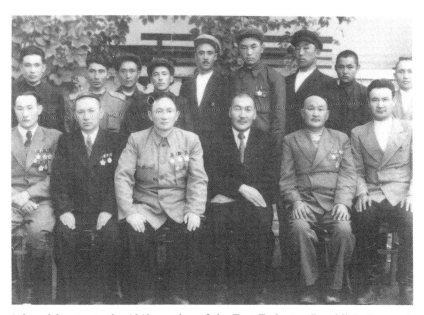

Ashan delegates to the 1949 meeting of the East Turkestan Republic's Economic Council in Yining [Gulja].

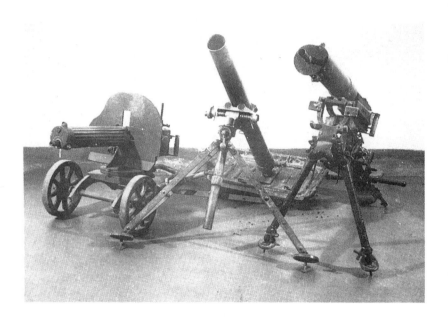

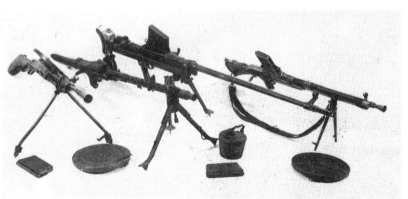

Weapons used in the military struggle in Xinjiang, 1944–1946

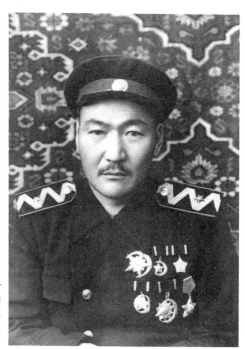

Delilhan Sukurbay, 1906–
1949. Kazak military leader of the
East Turkestan Republic and
member of the 1946 provincial coalition government.

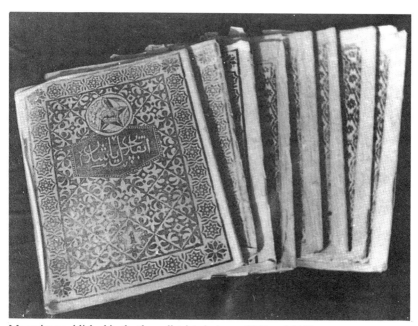

Magazines published in the three districts between 1945 and 1949

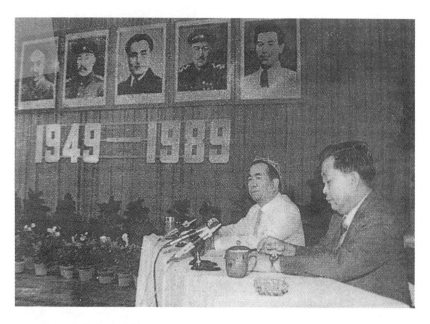

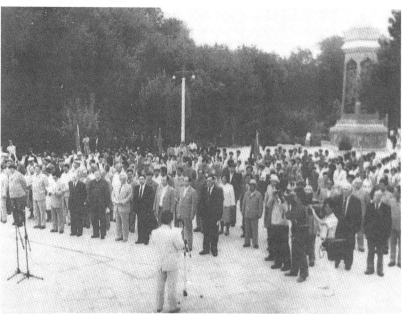

1989 memorial services at Yining [Gulja] for the leaders of the East Turkestan movement, now referred to as the Three Districts Revolution by the PRC government.

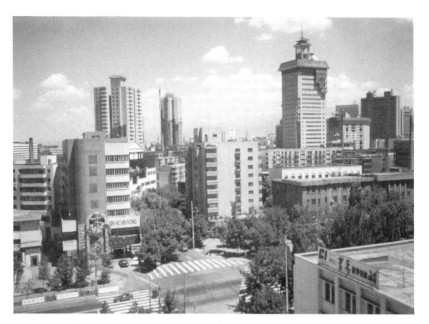

The new skyline of Urumqi, capital of the Xinjiang-Uyghur Autonomous Region
(Photograph by Linda Benson)

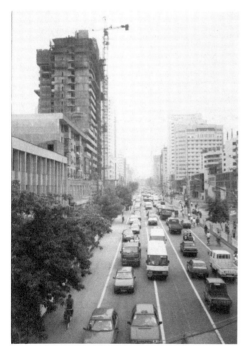

Traffic and major construction projects in downtown Urumqi, summer 1996 *(Photograph by Linda Benson)*

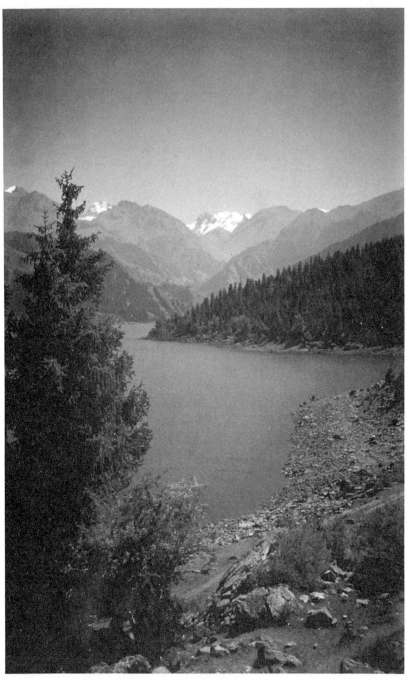

Tianchi Lake, a Kazak pasture area and tourist destination near Urumqi *(Photograph by Linda Benson)*

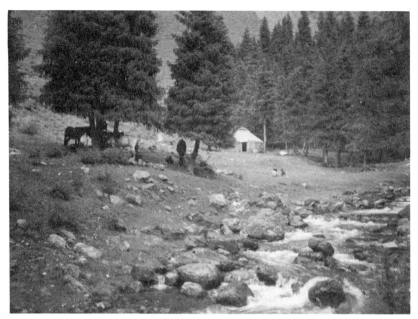

Kazak camp at Nanshan, south of Urumqi, summer 1996 *(Photograph by Linda Benson)*

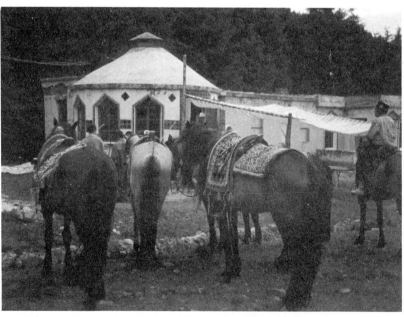

Kazak horses with traditional gear, outside a cement yurt at Nanshan, summer 1996 *(Photograph by Linda Benson)*

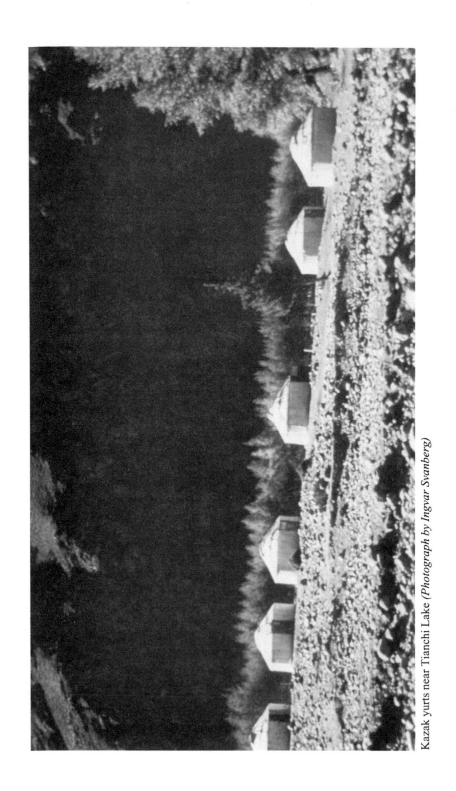

Kazak yurts near Tianchi Lake *(Photograph by Ingvar Svanberg)*

№	Cyrillic	№	Cyrillic
1	Аа	20	Оо
2	Әә	21	Өө
3	Бб	22	Пп
4	Вв	23	Рр
5	Гг	24	Сс
6	Ғғ	25	Тт
7	Дд	26	Уу
8	Ее	27	Уу
9	Ёё	28	Үү
10	Жж	29	Фф
11	Зз	30	Хх
12	Ии	31	hh
13	Йй	32	Цц
14	Кк	33	Чч
15	Ққ	34	Шш
16	Лл	35	Щщ
17	Мм	36	ъ
18	Нн	37	ы
19	Ңң	38	Іі
		39	ь
		40	Ээ
		41	Юю
		42	Яя

The Cyrillic alphabet intended for use among Xinjiang's Kazaks in 1956 varied somewhat from the Cyrillic form in use among the Kazaks of the USSR.

A	B	C	D	E	F	G
a	b	c	d	e	f	g
H	I	J	K	L	M	N
h	i	j	k	l	m	n
O	P	Q	R	S	T	U
o	p	q	r	s	t	u
V	W	X	Y	Z	Oı	Һ
v	w	x	y	z	oı	h
Қ	Ә	Ө	Ü	Ê		
қ	ә	ө	ü	ê		

A modified Latin alphabet was officially adopted for the Kazak language from the mid-1960s to 1980.

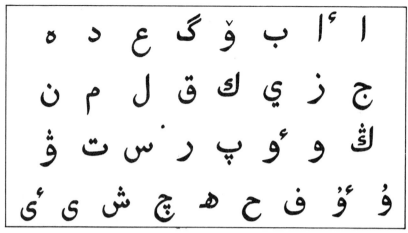

The contemporary Arabic alphabet used for writing Kazak in Xinjiang.

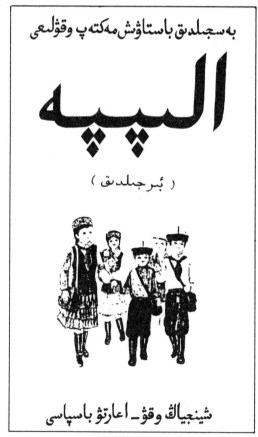

Cover of primary school text book in Kazak, published in Urumqi in 1986.

——— 6 ———

Kazak Culture and
Chinese Politics

In February 1997 the capital of the Ili-Kazak Autonomous Prefecture was torn by possibly the worst ethnic violence to erupt in Xinjiang since 1949. In what was described as "rioting" in the Chinese and international media, the Chinese police and military shot and killed a number of people in the streets of Yining. Hundreds were detained by the authorities in the aftermath, according to unconfirmed reports. The government declared martial law and closed the area to all outsiders except reinforcements for the Chinese military.[1]

Although the events of February 1997 may not be fully clear for some time, the incident marks a continuing pattern of conflict between Han and Muslim in the Kazak areas of Xinjiang. After a half century of CCP efforts, relations between Han and Muslims remain strained, periodically erupting into conflicts that fuel long-extant tensions. As the Beijing government continues with aspects of national and local policy that demand modification of Kazak cultural and religious practices, such tensions cannot be expected to abate.

In order to understand some of the complexities behind these repeated incidents, this chapter first examines areas of Kazak traditional culture that the government has attempted to influence or change since 1949; it then assesses Kazak response. In the process, we also look at ways in which Kazak society is currently changing; some changes are a result of government pressure, but others are a result of the Kazaks' own decisions to take advantage of new opportunities created in the region in the era of reform. Of greatest interest to both the government and the Kazaks are the following: Kazak language and literature; education; traditional nomadism, urbanization, and employment; religious

171

practice; and family planning. All of these areas are of special significance in that they are all aspects of a distinct Kazak identity. They are also areas in which the CCP has sought to intervene directly and to shape and control in varying degrees. In particular, practices that the party and government consider to be "backward" are viewed as obstacles to the modernization of China and are therefore targeted for eventual elimination.

While some manner of change would doubtless occur without Han intervention, regional authorities' attempts to quicken the pace of change have not only drawn Kazak resistance, but have also contributed to a heightened sense of Kazak identity and an increasing Kazak awareness of their minority status within Xinjiang. Further, as demonstrated below, attempts to change Kazak cultural practices feed the paradox of a growing sense of powerlessness among Kazaks on one hand and an increasing sense of ethnic pride on the other. In the 1990s, the presence of newly independent Kazakstan further complicates China's implementation of minority policy in Kazak areas that now border an independent Kazak state.

Kazak Language and Literature

After the death of Mao, the Chinese government's policy in cultural matters relaxed considerably. For minorities, this meant that attempts to control their written and spoken language lessened and that previous dictums were reversed. For the Kazak elite, the most important recent change occurred only in the 1980s when the Kazaks' right to use their traditional Arabic script was restored and publication using this form finally resumed.

For many Kazaks, however, the government's shifting language policy between 1949 and 1978 obstructed Kazak cultural expression. As the CCP sought to establish a clear policy on minority languages, it experimented with the introduction of first one written script and then another. The result was to divide the generations of Kazaks: People who were taught one form of the written language found themselves effectively illiterate when a shift was made to a new form. Whether this was the intent or not—and some believe it was intentional—the Kazaks found that the changes in written script divided them not only along generational lines, but also separated them from Kazaks in the USSR. To understand the situation more fully, we must start with a description of the language itself. Then we can address the attempted reforms since 1949.

Modern Kazak belongs to the so-called Kipchak languages, which are also referred to as the northwestern or Aralo-Caspian Turkic languages.[2] It is related to Kirghiz, Kazan Tatar, Mishar Tatar, Bashkir, Nogai, and Karaim as well as to some dialects of Uzbek—all of which are Turkic languages used today in Central Asia. During the nineteenth century, the elite of Central Asia used a common literary language, Chagatay, which was written in the Arabic script. At the end of that century, several spoken Turkic dialects of Central Asia were written for the first time, and these gradually replaced the increasingly archaic and elitist Chagatay form. Under the USSR, the policy was to emphasize the differences between these related languages. For instance, while many Western scholars regarded Karakalpak as a dialect of Kazak rather than as a separate language, the Soviets treated Karakalpak as a distinct language.

The Kazak language is very uniform, but some scholars also divide it into several dialects; the most important division is between the southern and northern dialects. The written language used in the USSR for the Kazaks was based on the northern dialect; China's Kazaks are considered to be speakers of the southern dialect.

Traditionally, Kazak was written in the Arabic script. In 1924 the USSR modified this form to better adapt to the Kazak sound system. In 1928, however, the USSR introduced a Latin script for the Kazaks. This was a move opposed by many Kazak intellectuals, but which was reportedly well received among the majority of the Kazak people, many of whom became literate for the first time in the new written form. In 1940, policy in the USSR shifted again, and a modified Cyrillic alphabet was introduced for all Turkic languages in the Soviet Union, including Kazak. This remained the official alphabet until the dissolution of the USSR in 1991.

In China before 1949, Kazaks used the Arabic script for their written language, while Kazaks in the USSR were changing first to the Latin and then to the Cyrillic form. After the 1949 revolution in China, discussion began on the most appropriate written form for China's own minorities; and clearly under Soviet influence, the government announced in 1956 that Xinjiang Kazaks would use the Cyrillic script. Uzbeks and Tatars living in China were to use the same Cyrillic form as their Soviet counterparts, while the Uyghurs, Kazaks, and Kirghiz were given a modified Cyrillic alphabet.[3]

Attempts to introduce the Cyrillic form among Xinjiang's Kazaks appear to have been only halfhearted. According to the proposed plans, it was expected to take some ten years before the new written forms would be fully utilized. But worsening Sino-Soviet relations interrupted this first attempt at language reform. There is little evidence to suggest that Kazak literature, for instance, was ever printed with the Cyrillic script in China, although it is quite possible that Kazak books printed in Cyrillic were imported for use in Xinjiang during the 1950s.

Just two years after the initial government announcement, the Cyrillic form was abandoned, a move prompted more by the Sino-Soviet split of 1958 than by linguistic considerations. Instead, the Kazaks were told to use the Latin alphabet, which was to be adapted for all languages in China. The new romanization for Chinese was the pinyin system, a Latin script that reformers believed would eventually replace even Chinese characters. Thus, all of China's citizens would share a single Latin-based alphabet, simplifying communication and language study throughout the country. Officially in Xinjiang the change was necessary because "the complicated written form [Arabic] now in use prevents the languages from meeting the needs of the swift development of socialist construction."[4]

In 1966, a massive campaign began to popularize the new forms for Kazaks and other Muslim minorities in Xinjiang. That same year, a newspaper in romanized Kazak appeared in the Ili area, along with periodicals in Uyghur and other Turkic languages, although the number of people able to read them must have been extremely limited.[5] Despite this seemingly eager embrace of yet another change, no immediate claims of great progress appeared in the press. During the course of the Cultural Revolution, which began the same year, language reform apparently languished while political struggles engulfed the region's Han population. Finally, in 1973, Chinese media reported that the new forms were now widely accepted by all the minorities in Xinjiang and that they were used in all primary and middle schools where instruction was in Kazak or Uyghur.

Experimentation with script reform finally culminated in a return to the Arabic script in 1981. Gradually, books in the Latin form were withdrawn from the bookstore shelves. New dictionaries, however, required time to prepare; in 1986 it was still easier to find a Kazak-Chinese dictionary in Latin script, such as *Kazakxa-Hanzuxa sözdik* (A Kazak-Chinese dictionary), than copies of the one Kazak dictionary using Arabic script, the *Han-Ha duizhao cihui* (A Chinese-Kazak bilingual dictionary). Ten years later, no Latin- or Cyrillic-script books in Kazak could be found in the regional capital's well-stocked bookstores.

By the 1990s, a fairly wide range of literature, texts, and reference works were readily available in Kazak. Newspapers, official announcements (pasted on the sides of buildings) and various notices all used the Arabic script as well as Chinese characters, suggesting that experimentation with script reform is now a thing of the past.

Increased literacy, discussed in the next section, has contributed to the demand for Kazak literature. In the past, the most important literary form was oral, which is the case with most of Central Asian literature. The main body of Kazak literature included epics, fairy tales, riddles, and songs. Some of this body of traditional Kazak literature began appearing in print for the first time in the 1980s. By 1986, there was a relatively large selection of Kazak language books available in Urumqi, including original Kazak works as well as translations of Chinese and foreign titles. Among the many works available in the 1990s are novels and poems, music, instruction manuals for animal husbandry, botany, forestry, medicine, agriculture, and so on. Younger readers are offered comics and children's books. Newspapers and magazines are published in Kazak as well as in the region's other major languages, and the Ili area carries news broadcasts on radio and television in the Kazak language.

Despite the satisfaction evident among Kazaks pleased by a return to the Arabic script, script reform was only one aspect of Chinese policy toward Kazak language and literature. Recent accounts by émigré Kazaks of the lives of leading Kazak literary figures in China assert that numerous such individuals have been detained by the Chinese authorities in Xinjiang over the years. These include the poet Tokhtarkhan Zhekebayev who was reportedly arrested in 1961 and subsequently executed. Another prominent author is Kazhykumar Shabdan, who was first detained during the Cultural Revolution. Upon his release, he wrote a book entitled *Crime,* which, according to Kazaks, helped expose the hypocrisy of the Chinese. This and other activities led to his re-arrest in 1986, whereupon he was sentenced to fifteen years in the laogai camps, a probable death sentence for a man in his late seventies. As the authorities release no information on such individuals, it is impossible to verify such reports. But it is clear that many people believe these stories to be true, and these tales of repression continue to feed a sense of resentment among many Kazaks.[6]

On the other hand, as noted earlier, traditional works of Kazak literature are being preserved by their publication and distribution in the region. The official attitude toward such works appears to be one of tolerance as long as the content does not include antigovernment messages. Kazak authors who accept these restrictions are also relatively free to write fictional works, providing an outlet for Kazak literary expression—albeit within limits imposed by the government.[7]

Education

In order to understand recent changes in education and its availability to Kazak people, we begin with a brief survey of Kazak education prior to 1949 and then turn to education under the current government.

Early in the twentieth century, education in Xinjiang was largely religious, with Muslim children usually attending school for religious instruction. Republican-era sources note that most Kazaks in Xinjiang were illiterate, with one Chinese source asserting that the illiteracy rate among Kazaks in the three northwestern border districts was over 80 percent as late as the mid-1940s. The actual level of literacy among the Kazaks remains uncertain, but figures on the number of schools and Kazak pupils suggest that a 20 percent literacy rate could be too low. For instance, figures for July 1938 indicate that Xinjiang had 275 Kazak schools, with a total of 14,322 pupils enrolled that year. It is possible that additional Kazaks attended the Uyghur schools, which numbered 1,540 and had an enrollment of 89,804 students. In addition, the region had one Hui school with forty-four pupils and twenty-four Mongol schools with 917 pupils.[8] In the Ili area, the city of Yining (Gulja) provided education in religious schools. A Tatar school had opened in 1941 offering a modern education, and the Russian school there was highly regarded.[9] In 1944, the year fighting erupted in the Ili Valley, the three northwestern districts along the USSR border reportedly had seventy-nine elementary schools, serving 6,200 pupils of all nationalities, according to a PRC source.[10] After 1944, the East Turkestan government based in Yining operated separate middle schools for girls and boys, as well as a school of science and technology.[11] By 1949 the number of elementary schools had increased

to 489 with 52,719 students; in addition, thirty middle schools reportedly served 1,610 students.[12]

The only tertiary education available in the region during the 1930s
and 1940s was at Xinjiang College, also called the College of Law and
Political Science, in Urumqi, where the quality of education was reportedly not very high. Whether that assessment is true or not, it did
provide higher education to local Muslims as well as to Han Chinese.[13]
Wealthier members of the local Muslim communities sought to edu-
cate their children outside the province; some Xinjiang residents received university-level education in neighboring republics of the
USSR, in Turkey, and in Europe.

Textbooks and printed materials remained in short supply in the
region prior to 1949, but some progress was made in this area, too,
despite the difficult circumstances. In 1941, a total of 81,900 textbooks
were published in Uyghur for elementary schools, and 15,400 were
published in Kazak, all in the Arabic script. Although the Chinese at
that time were a small percentage of the population, 109,000 texts were
published in Chinese the same year.[14]

Although the total numbers of Kazaks receiving formal education in
Xinjiang before 1949 was small, there was great respect for learning,
and a significant number of Kazaks were not only literate but possessed education beyond the elementary level. A Kazak elite with formal education had thus emerged by the eve of the PRC's founding.

After 1949, a major concern of the new government was to increase
the number of schools and to reduce illiteracy. Information on the
expansion of the education system in Xinjiang is summarized in table
6.1, which shows the increasing numbers of schools and students of all
nationalities. The jump in figures between 1956 and 1958 resulted, in
part, from the migration of Han into the region. Figures collected in
1990 reflect unexplained drops; for example, the number of senior
middle school students decreased by 3.8 percent, and junior middle-
school students fell 12.4 percent over the previous year.

Overall, incomplete figures for Kazak education since 1949 indicate a fairly steady increase in the number of Kazaks attending
schools at all levels. By 1982, the education level of the 725,130
Kazaks over the age of six included 2,547 people with a completed
university education, 41,599 who had attended upper middle school,
and 124,781 who had attended lower middle school. A total of
351,272 Kazak children attended elementary school. The number

Table 6.1

Total Schools and Students, 1952–1990

Year	Primary Schools	Students	Secondary Schools	Students
1952	—	307,000	—	16,162
1955	—	365,000	—	28,300
1956	2,000	400,000	71	—
1958	4,434	718,000	110	61,000
1960	4,500	957,000	44	—
1963	3,000	—	360	—
1973	10,051	1,292,000	854	450,000
1975	—	2,000,000	—	—
1983	8,261	1,941,000	2,123	873,657
1989	9,651*	1,842,100	—	893,200

Sources: Figures for 1952 to 1975 are based on Chinese newspaper reports. Figures for 1983 are from *Xinjiang-Weiwuer zizhiqu gaikuang* (Urumqi, 1985), 205. Figures for 1989 are from FBIS-CHI–90–135 (July 13, 1990), 50.

Note: No figures on education are available for the decade between 1963 and 1973.
*Figure is for primary and middle schools for all nationalities in 1988.

remaining illiterate or semi-illiterate was officially put at 203,448.[15]

Some Kazaks are moving to cities in order to receive a better education than available in rural areas. A small number of Kazaks attend Xinjiang University, where there are also a few Kazak professors teaching in various fields. Current policy gives preferential treatment to minority applicants to the university by allowing their admittance with lower scores than Han students. In Urumqi, intellectual leadership is provided by scholars at the Academy of Social Sciences, which employs Kazak scholars in several of its institutes, although the majority of scholars there and at other Xinjiang institutions of higher learning are Han. In addition, several Xinjiang Kazaks have received doctorates at various institutions in China, and a few have gone abroad to study in Russia, the United States, and Kazakstan.

By 1990, the average number of years of schooling for Kazaks in China was 6.45 years, above the average for all of China which was 6.26 the same year. It was also higher than the average of 5.29 years for all minorities in China. The Kazak illiteracy rate was reported as only 12.34 percent in 1990, indicating major strides in Kazak education.[16]

After the Cultural Revolution, minorities began attending tertiary institutions in small but growing numbers. By 1989, out of a total of 31,700 people attending schools of higher learning, 18,000 were minority nationalities, an increase over 1988. Colleges and universities in Xinjiang were enrolling 8,053 new students, an increase of almost 5 percent over the previous year. At the region's most prestigious school, Xinjiang University in Urumqi, 726 minority students enrolled in 1989, or 65 percent of the 1,118 new students enrolling that year. The number reportedly included Kazaks as well as other members of other minority nationalities, but no number for Kazak students was given. Overall, of the university's total student body of 5,063, 64.5 percent were of local Xinjiang minorities in 1989.[17] In addition, the government announced that 800 students from Xinjiang attended inland universities and college. Although no number was given, the 800 reportedly included a "large proportion" of minorities.[18]

Graduate studies remained available to only a few. In 1989, the region had a total of 339 graduate students, a decrease of 16 percent over the previous year. Only 74 new students enrolled in 1989, a 45 percent decrease over 1988—a drop not explained in government reports but possibly linked to demonstrations at many of the colleges and universities in the region in the late 1980s.[19]

The increasing education levels and expectations of a higher standard of living are important factors in the transition some Kazaks are choosing to make by moving into towns and cities. This change constitutes a major challenge to the Kazaks today, as the possibilities of urban life increasingly attract a new generation. As Xinjiang continues it rapid economic expansion and its policy of opening up to outside investment, more Kazaks will be faced with a choice between traditional herding and the newer lifestyle options in the cities.

Traditional Nomadism, Urbanization, and Employment

Underlying CCP policy toward nomads has been the view that these culturally and economically "backward" peoples need the guidance of their more advanced Han brothers in order to move toward a "modern" life. Translated into specific policy goals, this has meant concerted efforts to settle traditionally nomadic peoples like the Kazaks. The benefits to the Kazaks are stated explicitly in government pronouncements on the need for settling nomadic groups. These include such advantages as an overall higher income, access to better medical care, better education, and a more secure life than that provided by the traditional, unpredictable lifestyle of the nomad.

Given the lower income of herding areas and the shortage of medical and educational facilities in rural areas, life in villages or towns can indeed offer both greater economic security and a higher standard of living, just as government propaganda insists. But the alternative of settling has always been available to nomads in Xinjiang; the reason that Kazaks did not do so in large numbers is directly related to Kazak identity as nomads and to their economic reliance on animal herds necessitating less populous regions. Ending this lifestyle would mean a divorce from the traditional ways that mark Kazak society as separate and distinct from others. Thus the decision to settle is not simply a matter of security or better conditions: It implies a rejection of many elements considered fundamental to Kazak identity.

With the return to private herd ownership in the 1980s, the government increased its efforts to settle Kazaks. In 1990, an optimistic report by the government indicated that as of 1989, 56,000 herdsmen households had settled down, accounting for fully one-third of the total Kazak population in Xinjiang. In recounting why the herdsmen had decided to settle, the report read in part, "They were constantly threatened by natural calamities which would decimate their livestock. Moreover, their lifestyle made them economically and culturally backward."[20] In 1995, the government again reported that more herdsmen had settled permanently. Kazaks were reportedly relying on a combination of natural and man-made grassland to feed their animals and were penning their animals during the cold season in order to reduce losses.[21] However, there was no indication of the total number settled in this or in similar reports. If the 1990 report was accurate, in that year as many as two-thirds of the Kazaks continued in their traditional lifestyle, making them among the last of China's nomads.

Despite a lack of figures in reports such as these, other statistics indicate that some Kazaks have chosen to move to Xinjiang's growing urban centers (see figures on city populations and on growth of ethnic minorities in urban areas summarized in table 5.5). As of 1990, the region's overall urban population accounted for 31.9 percent of the total population of over 16 million.[22] Three urban areas boasted a population density of over 100 people per square kilometer: Urumqi,

Karamai, and Shihezi. All are predominantly Han industrial centers, closely linked by rail and by the region's main east-west highway. Incomes are substantially higher in the cities, as already noted. Statistics on the ethnic composition of towns and cities in Xinjiang are scarce, but figures summarized in table 6.2 show that as of 1991, Kazaks in the thousands are now urban residents. The largest group is in Urumqi, where the opportunity to double or triple the family income is a major attraction.

In 1992, population figures for Urumqi indicated a Kazak population of 42,218. Of these, 15,187 lived within the city limits while another 27,031 lived in Urumqi county.[23] Little data are available on this group, but in 1996 one of the authors was told that Urumqi had two elementary schools and one middle school providing education in the Kazak language, suggesting permanent relocation of families, not only working adults. All Kazak students study Chinese as a part of the schools' curriculum; with Chinese as their second language, their integration into the city's predominantly Han culture seems assured.

There are no systematic studies of Kazaks making what must be a difficult transition from rural to urban life. Moving into towns in Xinjiang necessitates cultural change and adaptation. Separated from the majority of Kazaks who remain in the three Kazak autonomous areas, new arrivals in cities like Urumqi must accommodate themselves to a population that is, at best, indifferent to their arrival. Everyday business with Uyghurs can be conducted in Kazak, which most Uyghurs can understand, but cities in Xinjiang are overwhelmingly Han Chinese, requiring arriving Kazaks and their children to master the Chinese language and adapt to a Chinese environment.

For some, proximity to the Han heightens awareness of their second-class status in China. For example, while their children may be able to enjoy an education in their own Kazak language, the Han schools are generally superior to minority schools. Moreover, Han students in urban areas have a clear sense of their own generally higher status, and, as in some other situations in which a minority receives preferential treatment, there is condescension toward young Kazaks who enter universities because they are admitted with lower scores than Han students.

Urban life is also expensive. While pay for some kinds of work is high, so are expenses. A small one- or two-room Urumqi apartment cost 600 yuan in 1996; the average salary for a young teacher or new government employee averaged 350 yuan the same year, making it necessary to have at least two wage earners in the family in order to just pay the rent.

As elsewhere in China, opportunities for employment can depend on connections. Interviews with minorities in the region during the 1980s and 1990s offered anecdotal evidence of high unemployment rates among young Muslims of all minorities, particularly in large cities like Yining. Confirmation of this perception came in 1990 from the regional chairman, Tomor Dawamat, who declared that unemployment among city and town youths was one of the most "outstanding" problems in Xinjiang.[24] Calling unemployment a "hot spot" in society, Dawamat indicated that measures would be taken to resolve the situation:

> The most outstanding problem today is unemployment among youth in cities and towns and a small number of enterprises stopping production. It is necessary to proceed from stabilizing the overall situation and actively implement the employment policy of the three-in-one combination of state enterprises, collectively owned plants, and self-employed workers, to actively open up the production sector, and to strive hard to develop the urban collective economy, rural enterprises, and the individual economy. It is necessary to increase employment and educate unemployed youth to help the country get over difficulties and take up difficult posts to temper themselves and mature. . . . It is absolutely not permitted to let them do whatever they think is right.[25]

In 1996, despite the priority that was supposed to be given to minority hiring, complaints over the difficulty minorities had in finding work continued. University-educated minorities interviewed in Urumqi that year felt themselves to be at a definite disadvantage when seeking employment, and the perception that Han are given the best positions remained relatively widespread among young Muslims of all ethnic groups.

While employment opportunities in cities were disappointing to Kazaks and other Muslims in the 1990s, the government announced in 1995 that out of 459,000 technical and professional workers in Xinjiang, 181,000 were minorities, showing a steady increase in the numbers of minorities trained for specialized, professional positions.[26] As Xinjiang has representatives of no less than forty-seven minority

Table 6.2

Kazak Populations in XUAR Cities, 1991

City	Kazak Population	Total Population
Urumqi	42,218	1,336,456
Karamai	8,286	210,208
Shihezi	3,297	533,710
Turpan	20	220,823
Hami	8,619	292,760
Changji	15,115	271,665
Kuitun	2,974	226,549
Yining	12,282	267,262
Tacheng	20,190	131,238
Altay	60,230	183,567
Bole	14,911	159,457
Korle	54	263,220
Aksu	22	397,517
Artush	26	171,374
Kashgar	37	230,397
Khotan	18	138,556
Total	188,299	5,034,759

Source: *Xinjiang nianjian 1992,* 40–41.

groups, however, it is impossible to speculate on how many of that number could be Kazak or, indeed, Muslims originally from Xinjiang.

Despite the problems experienced by Kazaks in Urumqi, Kazaks continue to move into towns and cities. Statistics from 1992 show that the largest numbers of urban Kazaks are in the cities of the Ili-Kazak Autonomous Prefecture, especially the traditionally Kazak areas of Altay and Tacheng—towns where the transition to urban life may be much easier than in Yining, the prefectural capital (see table 6.2). While the number of Kazaks in the capital constitute a small minority of only 4.6 percent, in the district capitals of Tacheng and Altay the percentage of Kazak residents was 15.3 percent and 32.8 percent, respectively. Kazak movement into urban areas will doubtless continue given the great disparity between rural and urban income. The encroaching agricultural sector, which has drastically reduced grazing lands for Kazak herds, will also play a role in moving numbers of Kazaks toward a settled life.

A possibly related problem emerging in both urban and rural areas, is alcohol abuse. In 1997, one émigré Kazak asserted that the authorities in China supported heavy drinking among the Kazaks by selling some of the cheapest vodka in the world at only two or three yuan a bottle.[27] Cheap wine and beer as well as kumiss are readily available, and public drunkenness is not unknown. High unemployment rates among Kazaks and other Muslim minorities, as suggested in Tomor Dawamat's 1990 speech, could contribute to an increase in alcohol abuse, although once again statistics on this problem are unavailable.

In Xinjiang of the 1990s, towns and cities remained divided into Muslim and Han sections, a division reinforced by language differences. Although many Han are second- or even third-generation residents in Xinjiang, few speak any local Turkic language; and many seem to share the first generation's contempt for "backward" ideas like religious belief and for "backward" cultures that need the guidance of the Han elder brother. Such attitudes increase the possibilities not only for cultural misunderstandings, but also for the kind of heightened awareness of deep-seated cultural differences that leads to violent confrontation.

Not only cultural differences divide Han and Kazak in urban settings. Further, Han assigned to border areas support the central government's agenda for rapid economic change and, along with it, the social change that brings the local population "up" to the level of the Han. Although clothed in the rhetoric of modernization, the underlying theme of "civilizing" the Kazak remains implicit in official government statements about the need for Kazaks and other nomads to pursue a settled life. This attitude is mirrored in the actions of Han officials assigned to work in minority areas. Ultimately, Kazak urbanization also reinforces an underlying goal of eventual assimilation of Kazaks and other minorities into the "higher" culture of the Hans.

Religious Practice and Education

In general, the attitude of the Chinese authorities in Xinjiang toward Islam reflects the legacy of Han-Muslim military conflict in the first half of the twentieth century, when religious leaders played important roles in efforts to secure autonomy or independence. After 1949, policy toward religion in Xinjiang followed the shifts in politics at the national level; official policy has thus ranged from tolerance to total repression, the latter most often linked to the suspected role of Islam in the region's continuing ethnic unrest.

The most consistent aspects of religious policy include attempts at co-opting religious clergy to support policy goals and, in times of civil disturbances, the detention of clergy suspected of "splittist activities." A concerted effort has been made to limit all religious education, although religious instruction once again became available in many parts of the region after 1980.

As noted in earlier discussions of the shifts in policy that accompanied the Great Leap Forward in 1958 and the Cultural Revolution from 1966 to 1976, religious practice, including the public observance of religious holidays and the availability of religious education, was severely restricted prior to the era of reform. Since then, there has been a return to the more lenient attitude of the 1950s—with members of the regional and local government appearing in public to honor the celebration of Kurban-bairam and Ramadan, for example. Xinjiang Muslims are again allowed to make the pilgrimage to Mecca. According to a government announcement in 1988, for example, 6,000 people from Xinjiang visited relatives abroad or made their religious pilgrimage between 1980 and 1987.[28] Although the government has not announced numbers of pilgrims by ethnic group, the opportunity to travel is very much limited by ability to pay. The official cost of 10,000 yuan, which the government considered the minimum amount a pilgrim would need to cover his or her expenses in 1988, would certainly exclude the vast majority of Kazaks, whose annual income in 1990 was still under 1,000 yuan a year.[29]

Money to assist in the restoring—and in some cases total reconstruction—of mosques damaged in the Cultural Revolution was another strong indication of a new governmental attitude after 1980. In a three-year period prior to 1988, the state council allotted special funds of an unspecified amount to maintain more than 13,000 mosques and religious centers. Further, thirty local Muslim leaders from Xinjiang were sent to the China Islamic Institute in Beijing for religious education, and a few were sent to Egypt at government expense in 1987–1988.[30]

Despite what appeared to be a new tolerance of religious practice, however, tension between the religious leadership and the government in Xinjiang has remained. For example, in 1990 Tomur Dawamat offered this statement on the region's religious policy:

[W]e must conscientiously implement the autonomous regional people's government's regulations on strengthening management of religious sites, implement the policy on religion, allow personages of religious circles and the religious masses to engage in normal religious activities and give splittists no opportunity to act. It is necessary to resolutely prohibit religious forces outside Xinjiang from meddling in religious problems in the region and resolutely oppose political schemes which take advantage of religion to create disturbances and advocate splittism.[31]

Concern over outside interference in religion is invariably linked to splittist activities, and it is this fear on the part of the government that has colored religious policy in Xinjiang. The Chinese media's references to national splittist activities "under the cloak of religion" are a reminder of the past power of religious leaders and an indication of the vulnerability of the region to pan-Islamic appeals. Although there is little evidence that such fears are justified, continued tight control over Xinjiang is, publicly at least, deemed necessary because of the existence of this possibility.

It is also because of the above concerns that religious leaders have been detained in numerous crackdowns in Xinjiang since 1980. When unrest occurs in one area of the region, the government response has been to detain religious leaders not only in the affected area but in other towns as well. After demonstrations or violent clashes, the government requires religious leaders to issue denunciations, calling on all people to desist from violence and to condemn antigovernment demonstrations of all kinds. The role of religion and religious leaders remains at the center of local tensions, which, as seen below, is also fueled by policies governing another important aspect of Kazak life—family size.

Family Planning

The one policy that has drawn continued, angry opposition from minority groups in the era of reform are the efforts to limit family size. China's one-child policy originally applied only to the Han majority, minorities being exempt on the grounds that most had only relatively small populations. Despite the high number of births per family among some minority groups, high infant mortality rates meant that the population growth rate among them remained low. Nonetheless, as early as 1982, Beijing decided that minorities should also be required to participate in the national campaign to reduce China's overall population. Autonomous areas could develop their own family-planning policies, but all were required to have some mechanism in place to implement family planning. By the middle of the 1980s, the Xinjiang authorities began to push the idea of the smaller family for minorities. The media featured stories emphasizing the advantages of smaller family size, linking that to a higher quality of life and to more opportunities for the one or two children born to a couple. Studies on continuing poverty in minority areas stressed the connection between low family income and having many children. In 1985, Xinjiang authorities announced that urban minority couples could have only two children. Minorities active in the CCP were to act as models and were informally urged to have only one child. Rural families could have as many as three or, in some instances, four children, depending on individual family circumstances. During the authors' visit in 1986, Kazaks and other Muslim groups in Xinjiang believed that stricter limits would soon be introduced. They uniformly opposed government interference in what was viewed as strictly a family matter.

Despite the official policy of discouraging large families and government statements that minorities have welcomed the new policy, Xinjiang had the highest birthrate of any area in China in 1987. The birthrate per thousand for all of China in that year was 21; in Xinjiang it was 27.3, with the next highest rate being the predominantly Muslim region of Ningxia with 25.1 births per thousand.[32] Xinjiang also led in the number of births beyond one child, reaching 45.2 percent of all births in 1988. However, Xinjiang also had the highest mortality rate 8.7 per thousand as opposed to 6.7 per thousand for all of China in 1988.[33] In these statistics, Kazak data are subsumed in those for all of Xinjiang; but from the author's personal observation in 1991 and 1996, it appeared that large families remained the norm for Kazak families in rural areas.

In 1988, tighter control over family size began in Xinjiang. In May 1988, new "provisional" regulations on birth control were announced. The region's guidelines reiterated the call for a two-child limit for urban minority couples and a three-child maximum for families in pastoral areas and rural villages. A report that year announcing the new regulations noted that the combined minority population in Xinjiang was now 8.63 million, or 61.39 percent of the region's total. The average rate of population growth in China was given as 1.84 percent, while that of national minorities was 2.63 percent, far higher than the national average.[34] Infant mortality rates were also high at 106 per thousand in 1982; some grassland areas in southern Xinjiang had infant mortality rates at alarmingly high rates of 150 to 200 per thousand.[35] Although the report left it to the reader to make the connection between infant mortality and the number of children, it implied that a smaller number of children would also decrease infant mortality.

Increasingly, the directives and pronouncements on the importance of minorities adhering to the new regional family-planning guidelines have been couched in terms of social progress. Tomor Dawamat, the Uyghur chairman of the Xinjiang-Uyghur Autonomous Region in 1988, was cited in a Xinhua report as saying that unplanned population growth "laid a heavy financial burden on each family but has also brought about social difficulties in education, medical treatment, transportation, goods supply, and employment." In his official view, "progress" for Xinjiang's people clearly relied on restricting family size because "without family planning, the mastery of modern science and technology, and raising labor productivity which we are now striving for will become empty talk."[36]

The 1988 appeal for strict adherence to the provisional guidelines was also directed at religious leaders. Dawamat noted that many Muslim countries practice family planning and that Xinjiang should not fall behind them. Religious leaders were asked to support the new policy, or least not to place obstacles in the way of the work.[37]

Another element also emerged in the 1988 birth-control campaign. In a June 1988 broadcast, Dawamat noted that population quality was another issue that ethnic minorities must not neglect.[38] While linking this idea to the threat of population increases outpacing food production in the region, the suggestion that more children somehow equated to lower quality people cannot have been very welcome among people like the Kazak, who view large families in a most positive light.

Statistics for 1989 indicated that despite government concern over family size and despite pressure that began at least as early as 1982 in urban areas, birthrates had not appreciably declined. According to a 1995 Chinese population study, the 1989 average birthrate for the whole country was 2.24, or 21.73 per 10,000, while the Kazaks rate was 4.74, or 39.51 per 10,000—the highest of any minority group in China.[39]

Further, projections based on population figures for 1982 through 1990 indicated that the Han had increased at a rate of 10.8 percent, while the minorities had increased at over three times that rate, 35.52 percent, in the same period. If this pattern continued, researchers warned, by the year 2000 minorities could constitute fully 10 percent of China's total population.[40]

Despite government efforts, large families have remained the preference of the Kazak population. Given the substantially rural locale of most Kazak families—still over 80 percent rural in 1992, according to government statistics—it is unlikely that the government can easily impose its ideal of a small family in Kazak areas. Since 1991, a complicating factor has been the existence of the Republic of Kazakstan, where the number of births per family remains high, possibly strengthening Kazak resistance to following Chinese birth-control regulations. Certainly, religious freedom and family-size restrictions are two key issues fueling the increase in violent, ethnic-based confrontation in the Kazak areas.

Ethnic Violence

Kazak concerns over the future of their cultural and religious life and dissatisfaction with conditions in the Kazak areas have led to demonstrations and to a series of violent confrontations with Han Chinese since 1980. Unsure of their collective future in a region that is viewed by the central government as a storehouse of natural resources and new economic opportunities for the Chinese state, Kazaks have joined together to express their objections to what are locally perceived as Han policies. Although some of the new policies have benefited Kazaks in the form of better incomes and improved access to education and medical services, these improvements have not drawn the majority of Kazaks into mainstream, Han-dominated society. Instead, increased awareness of their secondary status as minorities in their own country has made cultural issues especially sensitive—as can be seen in the various incidents that have marked the era of reform.

While detailed information on these emotionally charged events must be gleaned from a generally hostile Chinese press, several of the disturbances have been on such a large scale as to require at least partial accounts to be published in the Xinjiang media. The following summary of some of the worst ethnic violence in the region is based on Chinese media as well as on émigré accounts and interviews with Kazaks during visits to the region.

In 1980 and 1981 the Chinese press reported anti-Han demonstrations in the city of Kashgar. In the 1981 confrontation, a Uyghur worker was killed by a Han, and in the resulting anti-Han demonstrations two people were killed and many were wounded. The next reported protests came in the regional capital, Urumqi, in 1985, when what was described as a 2,000-strong Uyghur contingent of students from six universities and colleges demonstrated on December 19 against the central government's continuation of nuclear testing, in the southeastern part of the region, and against Han settlers in Xinjiang. From the press descriptions, it is impossible to ascertain whether Kazaks participated in these earlier demonstrations, but Kazaks soon staged their own such movements.

In April 1988 the first large-scale public demonstration occurred in the Kazak areas. According to Chinese press reports, students from six institutes of higher education in the Ili-Kazak Autonomous Prefecture went on strike over the publication of the novel *Distant White House*. Published in Shanghai by the Chinese Writers' Guild, the Kazaks believed that this book distorted their habits and customs and constituted an affront to the self-respect of the Kazak people.[41] According to the Hong Kong press, the novel featured a Kazak woman named Saliha who lived at the turn of the century and whose behavior was described as "fickle and lascivious." It was this depiction of a Kazak woman that led to the outcry against what the Kazaks saw as a distortion of their culture. The government evidently agreed; the book was pulled from circulation, but not before considerable damage had been done to ethnic relations in Yining.

On June 15, 1988, further demonstrations hit the region, this time once again in Urumqi. Reportedly touched off when an obscene remark about Uyghurs was discovered written on a door in a physics department lavatory, some 600 students marched in the streets, reportedly shouting slogans such as "drive out the Hans" and "we don't want to be ethnic slaves."[42] Although it is again unclear whether Kazak students participated, it is probable that Kazaks attending the university showed their sympathies with the Uyghur by participating in the marches.

Ili also witnessed further demonstrations in the summer of 1988. "Big and small character posters" reportedly appeared in public places in Yining as well as in Uyghur towns. This time the protesters included educated people, who declared, "The formulation that Xinjiang has been part of China since the ancient past lacks historical basis."[43]

Throughout the summer, reports of scattered demonstrations and protests continued in the press, at least one of which reported that Muslims openly accused the Han of racism.[44] Another probable cause of the 1988 unrest was the May 1988 announcement of new birth-control regulations, as discussed above.

In what was clearly an effort to refute minority arguments and assert the validity of the government's role in Xinjiang, Janabil, the Kazak regional deputy secretary-general for the party, visited the Ili-Kazak prefecture in August 1988 to deliver his message of nationality solidarity. In an address during his visit, he warned of a "small number of people at home and abroad with ulterior motives . . . deliberately undermining nationality solidarity so as to split the unit of the motherland." He used historical examples, from 60 B.C. onwards, to illustrate that Xinjiang was and always had been an integral part of China. Because of this long shared past, he asserted, the "slogan of 'Hans and minorities cannot do without each other' is true."[45]

The government's response to the demonstrations of 1988 also focused on outside interference in Chinese affairs. Wang Enmao, former head of the autonomous region who was serving as chairman of Xinjiang's advisory committee, responded with accusations against groups from beyond China's borders. Quoted in the *Shanghai Information Digest,* Wang stated that the biggest threat in Xinjiang was from "elements coming from outside to conduct acts of sabotage and separatism." He denounced the slogan of "independence of Xinjiang," suggesting that unknown forces were seeking to separate the region from China.[46]

Echoing Wang, the regional CCP Han Chinese chairman, Ba Dai, accused no less than seven foreign organizations of supporting splittist activities in Xinjiang. Among them was a group called the Kazak-Turk People's Charity Fund, as well as a number of groups using the name East Turkestan, harking back to the republic of the 1940s. As is the usual case with such reports, no specific names were mentioned in connection with these groups, nor were numbers of members or locations of activities.[47]

Evidently unconvinced by government statements or by Janabil's protestations of the need for a Han presence in Xinjiang, minorities clashed with Han again in November 1988. Hong Kong newspapers reported that Yining was among the Xinjiang cities where unrest was most serious, but few details were given.[48]

The unrest of 1988 continued into 1989, this time fueled by the publication in China of another book, *Sexual Habits of the Muslims,* which was considered an insult to all Muslims. Demonstrations against its publication and distribution erupted in all cities with major Muslim populations in northwestern China. In Urumqi, during May 1989, crowds of young Muslims attacked government and party buildings, smashed and burned cars, and injured some 150 police, public security officers, and office workers.[49] Students and professors also demonstrated at the Ili Teachers Institute and, like those in Urumqi, demanded withdrawal of the book from circulation. Government response in areas outside Xinjiang were relatively conciliatory, and the book was quickly withdrawn. In Xinjiang, however, the authorities crushed the demonstrations and subsequently arrested an unknown number of participants in Urumqi and Ili. The book was pulled from the shelves of bookstores but at a cost that can be computed only in unknown numbers of detainees.

In Ili, the government mobilized religious leaders in an attempt to respond to the demonstrations. Members of the Islamic Association's standing committee met with party and government officials to denounce all the demonstrators. A member of the association was quoted in the press as saying that the Ili demonstrations involved "savage acts" by "a gang of ruffians with ulterior motives." The book, it was suggested, was simply a pretext to carry out such violence in the name of protecting Islam.[50]

By the end of June 1989, the Urumqi courts had convicted ten individuals of plotting and stirring up the "May Nineteenth incident." Although the ethnicity of the individuals is not given in the government report on the sentencing, eight names were Muslim and two were Hui, or Chinese Muslim. Sentences ranged from one to fifteen years in prison; one individual was given a life sentence, and one was exempted from penalty on the basis that he was under eighteen at the time and had informed against the other "criminals."[51]

Outside of Xinjiang, Muslim students were also drawn into the events of "Beijing Spring" in 1989, when demonstrations occurred in many of the major cities of China demanding political and economic reform. According to one report, 3,000 Xinjiang students were among those protesting in Beijing in 1989.[52] The most famous of Xinjiang's student leaders was Erkesh Devlet, known in the Western press by the Chinese form of his name, Wuerkaixi. A Uyghur who subsequently fled the country in the crackdown that followed the June 4 incident in Beijing, he remains in exile.

One of the worst incidents of violence in Xinjiang occurred the following year in predominantly Uyghur Kashgar, where ethnic tensions erupted into what is known as the Baren incident. Officially, twenty-two people died in what the government labeled a counterrevolutionary movement. Many Muslims insist that the number of minorities killed was much higher, and hundreds were reportedly sent to prison in the clean-up that followed.[53]

The party moved quickly to forestall any carryover of the Baren fighting into the Ili area. Discussion sessions were held in all work units in the Ili district, and the unanimous results were immediately publicized: Minorities everywhere, the local Ili press reported, condemned the Baren "counterrevolutionary armed rebellion." On April 27, 1990, a television report stated that twenty members of religious circles in Ili praised the party's nationality policy and condemned the rioters, who were "guilty of carrying out the activities of splitting the motherland and undermining national solidarity under the cloak of religion."[54]

Between 1990 and 1994, there were scattered reports of bombings in cities throughout Xinjiang. In 1992, bombs exploded on public buses in Urumqi killing six people and wounding another twenty-six.[55]

In 1994 the Ili area was once more the site of ethnic violence. According to the Hong Kong newspapers, "instances of disturbance, riot and rebellion have occurred in Xinjiang since the end of September [1994], the most serious being in Urumqi, Yining, Kashi [Kashgar], Karamai, and Aksu." In Urumqi, the demonstrators demanded greater economic autonomy for the region: Slogans shouted by the crowds demanded that Xinjiang become a special economic zone. While Urumqi remained free of violence on this occasion, in Yining the demonstrations escalated into a major clash with authorities. According to the press, 500 people staged a sit-in on September 29; the crowd swelled to over 1,000 on September 30, some waving Kazak flags. The crowd demanded that local leaders meet with them. When they were refused, they attacked government buildings, fought with police, and burned vehicles. Reinforcements arrived and opened fire on the crowd. Twenty people were reported injured, including twelve public security personnel.[56] A curfew was imposed until October 8; no further information was available in the press.

Other cities also experienced demonstrations in 1994 that were violently repressed. In addition to Kashgar and Aksu, predominantly Uyghur cities, there were also work stoppages at Karamai. While the majority of workers there are Han, Karamai was also home to 8,286 Kazaks in 1992.[57] Demonstrations began in late September over work assignments and wages. According to a Hong Kong press report, "virtually all of the hard, heavy and dangerous oil well work is done by local minority nationalities." Demonstrators were also angered by a pay scale that gave administrators twice the wages of workers; in addition to higher wages, they also demanded better living conditions and benefits. They earned less in comparison to workers at other oil fields, they asserted; wages at Karamai were less than one-third those at Daqing, for example.[58] The government promised to investigate, but the outcome of the rallies and demonstrations in October 1994, which involved as many as 8,000 workers and their families, was not announced in the press.

Violence in Kazak areas increased in 1995. In Ili, Kazaks and other minorities once again launched demonstrations against government policy. According to Hong Kong reports, thousands of people participated that April in what were described as antigovernment riots. On April 24, demonstrators thronged the streets of Yining, growing from an initial 50,000 to an estimated strength of 100,000—including workers, teachers, and shopkeepers. Some slogans called for an end to communist rule in Xinjiang; even more worrying to the authorities were demands for an independent Kazak state in Ili or for the right for Ili prefecture to become a part of Kazakstan.

Towns previously not mentioned in the press gained media attention this time as well, indicating the spread of antigovernment sentiment throughout the Ili River valley. According to unconfirmed reports from Hong Kong, the towns of Zhaosu, Tekes, Nilka, and Qapqal all saw serious disturbances in the spring of 1995. In Zhaosu for instance, the military reportedly used armored cars to stop people from plundering government buildings and stealing guns from the local arsenal. In the fighting that broke out, some 200 people died and over 80 were arrested. In Tekes, army units fought with local Muslims, resulting in further deaths and arrests. The worst events reportedly occurred at Nilka and Qapqal, the former being the town where the 1944 fight against the Guomindang was launched. According to the Hong Kong press, a sit-in began on April 22 in this small town, and the authorities responded by cutting off power, water, and gas. When crowds surrounded and threatened government buildings on April 25, shouting demands that all Han leave Xinjiang, the police opened fire, killing an unknown number. The government declared a curfew beginning April 26, and 20,000 soldiers of the thirty-third and forty-first divisions arrived by air and by rail to enforce order and close off the region from the outside.[59]

While the above accounts remain uncorroborated, further incidents in nearby areas erupted in 1996, lending credibility to accounts of trouble in the Ili Valley the previous year. Xinjiang media reported a clash at Kuqa that led to the deaths of nine Muslims, described as splittists in the *Xinjiang ribao* in May 1996. The town of Kuqa is linked by road to the eastern end of the Ili Valley; the road was closed for a period of time following the violence in May, which also claimed the lives of men in the Chinese military and local police.[60]

Possibly the worst incident in Kazak areas since 1949 occurred in February 1997, involving an unknown number of Kazaks and Uyghurs who reportedly clashed with local police and military units. As noted at the beginning of this chapter, the violence in Yining left an unknown number of people dead in the city's streets and many more under arrest. If true, this would be the worst incident in the region since 1949.

Yining has a relatively small Kazak population, less than 4 percent of the total in 1991. Unconfirmed reports say that the majority of those involved in the street fighting in 1997 were young Uyghur men and women protesting against the actions of the predominantly Han Chinese police and military. Nonetheless, the city is the center of government for China's single largest Kazak area. Imposing martial law and moving in large number of troops meant that regardless of the extent of Kazak participation, Ili Kazaks were certainly affected by the Chinese crackdown. In addition to a curfew, the city was closed to all but local residents, and the international border with Kazakstan was closed for five days.

As if to emphasize the Ili unrest and keep the Xinjiang region in the public eye, the February disturbances at Yining were followed by bus bombings in Urumqi on February 25, the day of Deng Xiaoping's funeral in Beijing. Two weeks later, similar bus bombings occurred in Beijing itself, seriously injuring at least eight passengers.[61] The Chinese press quickly labeled these incidents the work of Muslim separatists and terrorists and the authorities promised swift punishment for the perpetrators. Reports of detention and interrogation of Uyghurs all over China quickly spread in Xinjiang and among Xinjiang residents abroad.

Because there is no independent media in the region, rumors in Xinjiang have retained great power, as in the pre-1949 years, allowing even relatively small groups to use existing tensions to their benefit as stories circulate and possibly amplify the numbers and the seriousness of disturbances. Stories of outside assistance and of the existence of highly organized and well-funded separatist movements are repeated on the grapevine. Government action to suppress or counter such rumors appears, instead, to give them greater credibility, making them a factor in continued unrest.

Although the exact details and extent of the incidents described above have yet to be fully disclosed, accounts appearing in the Chinese media nonetheless make it clear that the Ili area has been the site of serious disturbances for nearly a decade. The situation constitutes a significant challenge to the Chinese authorities, who are facing a much more politically aware Kazak population than at any previous time. The existence of neighboring Kazakstan and its future relations with China as well as with China's Kazak population are new factors in the complicated and tense situation in the Xinjiang of the 1990s. Kazakstan may hold the key to future ethnic relations in northwestern China, as the Kazak areas of Xinjiang increasingly orient themselves toward Central Asia rather than toward Beijing.

—— 7 ——

Kazakstan and China's Kazaks in the Twenty-First Century

Since 1978, the Kazak areas of northwestern China have been most deeply influenced by two powerful forces: internal Chinese policy, which increasingly expects conformity with national agendas by minorities like the Kazaks, and international developments, including the establishment of the independent Republic of Kazakstan in 1991. Previous chapters have charted some of the internal changes in Kazak areas of China, leading up to the more rapid pace of change in the 1990s. In this chapter we focus on the impact of the Republic of Kazakstan, which, for the first time in 300 years, offers Kazaks dispersed throughout the world an independent, Kazak-administered homeland.

China and Kazakstan before 1991

Beginning in 1949, relations between China and the neighboring Kazak Soviet Socialist Republic were uneasy at best. An important element of this unease was the role played by the Soviet Union in Xinjiang during the first half of the twentieth century—in particular, its support of the East Turkestan Republic and its Muslim-led government. Although the CCP leadership may have been unsure of the exact nature of the USSR's involvement, it shared the misgivings of the Guomindang. Thus, despite superficially good Sino-Soviet relations and the Treaty of Friendship and Alliance signed by the two communist powers in 1950, the new government in Beijing remained distrustful of Soviet intentions in the northwest. As this distrust deepened into an ideological rift, relations deteriorated, although local Muslims continued to cross the border into the neighboring Kazak republic. By 1958, however, the treaty was a dead letter, and joint Sino-Soviet exploration and exploitation of Xinjiang's natural resources halted. The border between the two was closed by 1962, effectively cutting off all legal contact between Kazaks on either side of the border.

During the Cultural Revolution the Kazak-Xinjiang border was the site of armed clashes, as already recounted. Border incidents rocked the region in 1968 and again in 1969, bringing to a halt the Cultural Revolution in Xinjiang. Although the shooting ended in 1969, a state of "cold war" began; the Soviets used radio broadcasts into the region in continued attempts to discredit the CCP and its policies, appealing to Uyghurs and Kazaks to oppose the Chinese communist line. Émigré Kazaks and Uyghurs on the Soviet side of the border were drawn into these activities, providing round-the-clock attacks on the PRC over the airwaves through the 1970s.

It is understandable then that although China's era of reform began in 1978, Xinjiang's own "opening to the outside world" began slowly. As late as 1986, a number of sensitive border areas still remained closed to western visitors, including the Ili Valley.[1] Despite this, contacts between families separated since 1962 resumed in the 1980s. Initially, such travel was not made easy by the Chinese, who required that Xinjiang residents first make the expensive and time-consuming journey to Beijing to get a passport before returning home to make the relatively short and cheap journey from Xinjiang into the Kazak republic.

As late as 1989, however, the Chinese remained wary about people-to-people contacts. When a cultural festival was held that year in Almaty, Kazak bards (*aqin*) from all over the Kazak republic as well as from other Soviet republics and Mongolia participated, but no Kazaks from China attended. During the festival, a blind bard from Dzhambul engaged a female Kazak bard from Mongolia in a singing contest, a traditional form of musical dialogue that was used as a vehicle for veiled criticism during the Stalinist period. Improvising lyrics, he sang, "She has come all the way from Mongolia to perform here, but why do we not have any participants from China? Haven't the authorities opened up the border to Ili so that the Kazaks will be able to come here?" The following year, a Kazak cultural group was allowed to perform in Urumqi, but such contacts have remained limited despite the official policy of "opening up to the outside world."[2]

Kazakstan and China Since 1991

The Soviet Union's collapse in 1991 returned to Kazak hands the authority they had lost to the Russians over a hundred years earlier. On December 16, 1991, Kazakstan declared itself an independent republic; five days later it joined the CIS, of which it remains a member. In early January 1992, the new Republic of Kazakstan applied for membership in the UN. That same month it received official recognition from the United States, the PRC, the European community, and other nations.

One of the new policies of the Kazakstani government was to ease the way for Kazaks to return to Kazakstan. An exemption from taxes for the first two years, and assistance with housing and land were intended to aid Kazaks wishing to settle in the new Kazak state. Despite such assistance, the number of returning Kazaks has not been high. Indeed, more Russians have arrived than Kazaks. According to a recent study by Martha Brill Olcott, the Kazakstani government reported that more than 100,000 Russians arrived in 1992, while only 70,000 Kazaks arrived in the same year. The number of returning Kazaks dropped in 1993 and again in 1994, matched by a decline in Kazakstani interest in encouraging such immigrants, given the financial demands of resettling the newcomers.[3]

One of the first agreements between Kazakstan and China concerned the important issue of Xinjiang Kazaks returning to Kazakstan. In 1992, both governments signed an agreement on this issue, easing the way for the settlement of Xinjiang Kazaks in Kazakstan.[4] Although no data are available on the number of Xinjiang Kazaks who have returned to Kazakstan since the agreement, interviews with Kazaks in Urumqi in 1996 suggest that while initially a substantial number had hoped to emigrate, enthusiasm had already declined. Some would-be immigrants had already returned to Xinjiang because of the economic situation in Kazakstan.

The movement of Kazaks into Kazakstan is only one matter of interest to the governments of China and Kazakstan. Equally if not more important have been trade issues. Both sides have chosen to build on existing plans for economic relations. In 1989, the two had already signed an agreement covering economic and technological cooperation for the years 1989–1995. That summer a delegation from Xinjiang, led by the vice-chairman of the autonomous region, Hederbai, visited the Kazak socialist republic to attend the Xinjiang Export Commodity

Sample Fair, an event sponsored by the Xinjiang International Economic Cooperation Corporation in Almaty. During this visit, the Xinjiang delegation signed additional trade agreements that, according to the Xinjiang radio service, involved thirty-eight economic and technological projects valued at over 40 million Swiss francs.[5] In the summer of 1989, various issues related to the opening of the rail link between the USSR and China were also resolved, paving the way for the final phase of work to complete the railroad line.[6]

The dissolution of the USSR did not impede any of these arrangements, which simply shifted from the Kazak Soviet Socialist Republic to the Republic of Kazakstan. With Kazakstan's independence in December 1991, arrangements were quickly made for high-level visits to discuss cross-border trade and other issues. In 1992, Kazakstan's prime minister, Tereshchenko, paid an official visit to Beijing and signed an agreement for increased economic cooperation, laying the groundwork for subsequent agreements and a series of state visits by the Kazakstani president, Nursultan Nazarbaev.

Nazarbaev won Kazakstan's first presidential election, held on December 1, 1991. In a national referendum in April 1995, his term was extended to the year 2000.[7] A member of the Kazak's Ulu Juz, which had dominated politics in Kazakstan throughout the Soviet era, Nazarbaev has sought to maintain a largely secular state, with economic ties to all the neighboring countries. Foremost among these is Russia, still the major trading partner of Kazakstan seven years after independence.

China, however, is Kazakstan's most important non-CIS trading partner. In 1992, trade with China accounted for 20 percent of Kazakstan's exports and 42 percent of its imports. Imports from China via Xinjiang include some of Xinjiang's agricultural products such as sugar, corn, wheat, and fruit, as well as animal products such as horses, live and frozen sheep, and cattle. Manufactured products from China sold to Kazakstan include clothing, shoes, electrical goods such as radios, tape recorders, VCRs, and electric fans, and construction materials.[8]

To encourage the growth of trade with Kazakstan, the Xinjiang regional government has held several trade fairs. The first was in September 1992, when the Urumqi Frontier and Local Economic Relations and Trade Establishment Fair opened in Urumqi. Representatives from Kazakstan, Russia, Japan, Pakistan, Mongolia, and Hong Kong attended the fair, and a number of contracts were signed.[9] A second fair

was held in 1993. By 1994, Xinjiang and Kazakstan had signed papers for 136 joint ventures and other forms of investment.[10]
Overall, trade via the new ports of entry on the Xinjiang-Kazakstani border expanded tremendously in the first five years. Six of the new ports are by road: They include the three Altay district ports of Ahitubek (Aheitubieke), Jimnai (Jimunai), and Baktu (Baketu); three more are in the Ili area, Korgas (Ke'erguosi), Dulata (Dulata), and Muzart (Muza'erte). The most important route, however, is the railway link that crosses the Chinese-Kazakstani border at Alataw (Ala Shankou), in the Bortala-Mongol Autonomous Prefecture. (Alataw appears on many maps as the Dzungarian Gates, through which the Mongols stormed on their way to world conquest in the thirteenth century.) Over 700,000 tons of goods passed through Alataw in 1992, the largest of any of the fifteen ports then open. The value was estimated at nearly 80 million U.S. dollars the same year.[11] By 1994, the value of trade through the fifteen ports was put at 570 million U.S. dollars.[12] Cross-border trade continues to attract Han and Muslim traders to the area, all intent on taking advantage of the new opportunities to make money in the consumer-goods-poor countries of the CIS. Business is done on various levels, some being the province of peddlers and individual traders, who find a ready market in Kazakstan for consumer goods ranging from televisions and VCRs to inexpensive everyday household items. Construction workers and truck drivers from China have also found new opportunities in Kazakstan as well, to the extent that some Kazakstani and Kirghiz have protested over a "Chinese invasion" of workers and traders during the mid-1990s.

Kazak Nationalism: China's Next Challenge

While economic contacts are being pursued with some vigor by the Chinese government and by enterprising traders of all kinds, Chinese authorities must also deal with an independent and nationalistic Kazak state currently undergoing a national cultural revival. At issue is the need for China to follow policies that forward China's goals of economic expansion while at the same time forestalling a rise in nationalism among its own Turkic Muslims and, most importantly, among the million-strong Kazak population in Xinjiang. To this end, Kazakstan's first deputy prime minister, Nigmatzhan Isingarin, who accompanied Nazarbaev on a state visit to China in 1995, publicly announced that among other matters covered by a September 13, 1995, joint communiqué, the two governments agreed to a clause concerning "anti-national splittism." In order to maintain stability and peace along their borders, both sides agreed not to allow any separatist activities on its territories.[13] These agreements were publicly reconfirmed in 1997 on the heels of the disturbances in Yining.[14]

However, even with both governments cooperating to limit the amount of political organizing done within their borders, the cultural revival underway in Kazakstan will be difficult to contain. Symbols of Kazak national identity are very popular and are vigorously promoted in Kazakstan. The use of Kazak, not Russian, as the national language is a daily reminder of Kazak national pride, despite the wide use of the Russian language among the educated. The new constitution, for example, decreed that the president must be a Kazak speaker. Russian street and place-names have disappeared, as in other newly independent states—contrasting with Xinjiang, where Chinese place-names still take precedence over Kazak forms in some areas. In Kazakstan, there are celebrations for traditional Central Asian holidays and observance of festivals such as the Persian New Year, Nauriz (Navrez Meram), as well as all the Muslim holidays. Kazakstani intellectuals have embraced a return to a Kazak identity, even as efforts to recapture, or in some instances recreate, a Kazak identity continue to be the focus of public discussion.

An important element of cultural revival is the ongoing effort to rewrite Kazak history, free of the restrictions imposed by Soviet Marxism. Scholars at the Kazakstan Academy of Sciences in Almaty are not only interested in writing the history of Kazaks in Kazakstan, but are also examining the history and status of Kazaks outside their country, the Kazak diaspora. The Kazakstani Soros Foundation, for instance, is translating Western scholarly books about Kazaks in China and Turkey into the Kazak language in an effort to expand knowledge of other Kazak communities as well as to familiarize Kazaks with Western social scientific methods.

Of special interest to Kazakstani scholars are Xinjiang's Kazaks, many of whom have close relatives in Kazakstan. As China was closed for an entire generation, events and personalities in this century have drawn the attention of scholars seeking to understand fully the history of their compatriots in China. Events that remain highly sensitive in China, such as those occurring in the period of the East Turkestan

Republic (1944–1950) are of great interest, as is the fate of those Kazaks who fled Xinjiang and resettled in Turkey in the early 1950s. Descendants of the latter group are also anxious to reexamine the events in which their parents and grandparents participated. With contact between Kazakstan and Turkey expanding, it is likely that Kazakstani publications on such sensitive matters may reveal versions of events not acceptable in China. As research on such topics proceeds, the "open border" between China and Kazakstan may become an avenue of information and new interpretations unwelcome to the PRC authorities. Regardless of agreements limiting political activity on each other's soil, information that contradicts the government line can undermine China's slogan of "*minzu tuanjie*" (nationalities' solidarity) in far more dramatic ways that the recent demonstrations in the Ili area have.

Indeed, repeated disturbances in the Ili area since 1991, as recounted in chapter 6, suggest that Kazaks in Xinjiang are already being directly or indirectly influenced by Kazakstan's independence and its fostering of national Kazak pride. Many of the younger generation of Kazaks in China understand the risk they are taking when they join in demonstrations and public protests. Their willingness to take to the streets despite the presence of military units and paramilitary groups like the PCC—not to mention the harsh sentences meted out to anyone contravening regulations on public order—is one indication that Beijing will need to do more than rely on economic gains to satisfy Kazak desire for a greater voice in local issues.

The Environment: A Pan-Kazak Concern

While there is little indication that Kazaks in Kazakstan or Xinjiang are interested in either pan-Turkic or pan-Islamic movements, intellectuals and activists from both areas are united on issues that transcend national borders. The most important of these is pollution caused by nuclear testing in Central Asia. Both Xinjiang and Kazakstan were used for nuclear testing by their respective governments. The first test in Kazakstan occurred on August 29, 1949; weapons were tested above ground until 1963, after which time tests were moved underground. Both countries exploded numerous nuclear devices at guarded testing sites, from which radioactive leakage has caused severe environmental damage. In the 1980s people began to realize that the tests led to genetic damage and a reduction in the effectiveness of human immunity systems. International movements helped to organized antinuclear groups, which began to stage protests in Kazakstan before 1991.

In 1988, members of the Nevada-Semipalatinsk-Lop Nor Anti-nuclear Movement demonstrated against the continued underground testing of nuclear weapons in Kazakstan and Xinjiang, drawing international attention to the issue of nuclear testing in Central Asia. Demonstrations in Kazakstan continued until 1991 when Nazarbaev closed the test sites there. In China, however, testing continued underground until 1996, when the PRC finally signed the international nonproliferation agreement, even while it maneuvered to reserve Chinese rights to resume testing in certain circumstances.

The heritage of nuclear testing is only one element in the region's environmental degradation. In Kazakstan, both Almaty, the national capital, and Karaganda, a major city of northern Kazakstan, suffer from severe air pollution as a result of industrial discharge. Industrial pollution and unsafe disposal of chemical and other wastes has resulted in eastern Kazakstan's being designated an ecological catastrophe zone, a label which has become alarmingly common in areas once part of the USSR. On the Chinese side of the border, exile Kazak groups assert that grassland in the Altay area has been destroyed by both acid rain and pollution. Other exile organizations claim that because of such contamination of the environment various forms of cancer are increasing in Xinjiang. For example, the rate of leukemia in Xinjiang reportedly increased seven times between 1975 and 1985; the incidence of other forms of malignancies such as esophageal and vaginal cancer are also reportedly on the increase, as are birth defects and complications in pregnancy and birth. It is probable that the latter may be linked to the high levels of infant mortality mentioned in chapter 6. As far as is known, these issues have not yet been discussed by representatives of China and Kazakstan, despite local concerns.[15]

Conclusion

Ultimately, the Kazaks of the twenty-first century will face the same geopolitical reality they face in the twentieth. China's rapidly growing wealth, its vast population, and its military power will allow it to dominate Central Eurasian politics. Kazakstan, for all its vast size and as yet untapped natural resources, has only 16 million people, roughly the same population as the Xinjiang region itself. Even if Kazakstani authorities had the desire to assist the Kazaks in China in their struggle for greater autonomy, they would have to deal with a China as capable of saying "no" to minority demands for greater regional autonomy as to the diplomatic overtures of other great powers. Although Kazaks in China may see Kazakstan as providing a means to pressure China for greater freedoms or, at least, for exemptions from some policies, the success of this pressure remains unlikely for the foreseeable future.

This does not mean, however, that Chinese economic and military power will be able to quiet increasingly restive minorities like the Kazaks or to resolve the challenge of being a multiethnic state in an era of rapid international communications. Xinjiang is no longer the isolated outpost it was at the time of the Qing, and any effort to keep outside influences from shaping events there is not likely to succeed.

As the governments of Kazakstan and China gain experience in international affairs, their approach toward—and understanding of— the issues raised by the presence of Kazaks on their long-shared border will doubtless undergo modification. In the meantime, Kazaks in both states have new opportunities to understand and build on their collective past, as they reestablish contacts with relatives and friends across the border. Although Kazakstan's government may not be able to use political or military clout to influence China's minority policy in the next century, it can and will provide a cultural model for Kazaks all over the world, reviving and recreating a distinctive cultural tradition. This newly invigorated pride in Kazak identity will also provide a challenge to both governments as they seek to maintain stability in this historically volatile corner of the globe.

Notes

Notes to the Introduction

1. Patrick Conway, "Kazakhstan: Land of Opportunity," *Current History* (April 1994), 167.
2. For further information on Kazaks in Mongolia, see Ingvar Svanberg, "Vilken roll spelar den Kazakiska diasporan?", *Centralasien-gamla folk soker ny vag* (1995): 15–25; and Peter Finke, *Nomadismus der Kasachen in der Westmongolei*. Unpublished thesis, Freie Unversität Berlin, 1995.
3. Audrey Shalinsky, *Central Asian Emigres in Afghanistan: Problems of Religion and Ethnic Identity* (1979), 11.
4. For further information see Halife Altay, "Hur Dunyada Turkistan Muhacirleri," [The Free World's Turkestani Refugees] *Turkeli* (1978), 5:16–22.
5. Ingvar Svanberg, "Etniska och sprakliga minoriteter i Iran," in Hans Backman, ed. *Inte bara sh'ia. En bok om Iran och dess minoriteter* (1992), 103–125.
6. For detailed discussion, see Ingvar Svanberg, *Kazak Refugees in Turkey: A Study in Cultural Persistence and Change* (1989).
7. Ingvar Svanberg, "Vilken roll spelar den Kazakiska diasporan?" *Centralasien-gamla folk soker ny vag* (1995), 15–25.

Notes to Chapter 1

1. Anonymous, *Xinjiang: The Land and the People* (1989), 8.
2. A Chinese publication states that the translation for the Uyghur name "Takla Makan" is "go in and you won't come out." See Anonymous, *China: A Geographical Sketch* (1974), 44. However, Uyghur scholars contend that it is an old form of the words for "Grape Arbor." Personal communication with Dr. Dolkun Kamberi, L. Benson.
3. E. M. Murzayev, *Prirode Sin'czjana i Formirovanie pustyn' Central'noj Azii* (The Nature of Sinkiang and the Formation of the Deserts of Central Asia) (1966) 350–351.
4. Theodore Shabad, *China's Changing Map: National and Regional Development, 1949–1972* (1972), 346.
5. On Uyghur history from a Chinese viewpoint, see Ma Jiasheng, Cheng Suoluo, and Mu Guangwen, *Weiwuer shiliao jianbian* (A concise edition of historical materials on the Uyghurs) 2 vols. (Beijing: 1981). For an English account of Uyghur ethnogenesis, see Chen Chao, "A Summary of Discussions on the Origin of the Uygur People in Xinjiang," *Social Sciences in China* 3.2 (1982):

18–26, and Geng Shimin, "On the Fusion of Nationalities in the Tarim Basin and the Formation of the Modern Uighur Nationality," *Central Asian Survey* 3.4 (1984): 1–14. For an assessment of these views and alternative interpretations, see Linda Benson, "Contested History: Issues in the Historiography of Inner Asia's Uighurs," in Michael Gervers and Wayne Schlepp, eds. *Toronto Studies in Central and Inner Asia,* no. 2 (1996), pp. 115–131.

    6. W. Barthold, *Turkestan down to the Mongol Invasion* (1958), 386.

    7. Tsing Yuan, "Yakub Beg (1820–1977) and the Moslem Rebellion in Chinese Turkestan," *Central Asiatic Journal* 11 (1961): 134–167.

    8. Owen Lattimore, *Pivot of Asia* (1950), 50.

    9. Wen-djang Chu, *The Moslem Rebellion in Northwest China, 1862–1878* (1966).

    10. Lattimore, *Pivot of Asia,* 140.

    11. On nineteenth-century Xinjiang, see K.B. Warikoo, "Chinese Turkestan during the Nineteenth Century: A Socio-economic Study," *Central Asian Survey* 4.3 (1985): 5.

    12. "Survey of Shanghai Youth in Xinjiang," *China Daily* (November 28, 1986).

    13. FBIS-CHI–90–250 (Foreign Broadcast Information Service-China). December 28, 1990, 54.

    14. On Chinese Muslims, see Françoise Aubin, "Chinese Islam: In Pursuit of Its Sources," *Central Asian Survey* 5.2 (1986): 73–80, and Dru Gladney, *Muslim Chinese: Ethnic Nationalism in the People's Republic* (1991).

    15. FBIS-CHI–90–250 (December 28, 1990), 54.

    16. Ibid.

    17. *Xinjiang nianjian 1992* (Xinjiang Yearbook 1992), 40.

    18. FBIS-CHI–90–250 (December 28, 1990), 54.

    19. C. Mannerheim, "Across Asia from West to East in 1906–1908," *Societe Finno-Ougrienne, Travaux ethnographiques VIII,* vol. 1 and 2 (1990), 210; Stanislaw Kaluzynski, *Die Sprache des mandschurischen Stammes Sibe aus der Gegend von Kuldscha* (1977), 7.

    20. FBIS-CHI–90–250 (December 28, 1990), 55.

    21. Kaluzynski, 39.

    22. E.N. Nadzhip, *Modern Uigur* (1971), 13.

    23. Geng Shimin, "Die Turksprachen Chinas und Ihre Erforschung," *Materialia Turcica* (1988): 12–19.

    24. For details on Xinjiang's Russian minority, see Linda Benson and Ingvar Svanberg, "The Russians in Xinjiang: From Immigrants to National Minority," *Central Asian Survey* 8.2 (1989): 97–129.

Notes to Chapter 2

    1. Denis Sinor, *The Cambridge History of Inner Asia* (1990); Otto Maenchen-Helfen, *The World of the Huns* (1973).

    2. See Su Beihai, *Hasakezu wenhuashi* (The cultural history of the Kazak nationality) (1989), and other works from China listed in the bibliography.

    3. Martha Brill Olcott, *The Kazaks* (1987), 4.

4. See Marjorie Mandelstam Balzer, *Shamanism: Soviet Studies of Traditional Religion in Siberia and Central Asia* (1990).

5. On issues in the writing of minority history, see Stevan Harrell, ed., *Cultural Encounters on China's Ethnic Frontiers* (1995).

6. See, for example, Su, *Hasakezu wenhua shi.*

7. Olcott cites Soviet sources saying that Giray's son Buyunduk ruled first, from 1480 to 1511. Olcott, 8.

8. This people has also been called the Eleuth, Oelot, and Oirat. The Oyrats' main tribes in the 1600s included the Khoshuts, Turguts, and Choros: The Choros tribe included the subtribes of the Derbet, Khoit, and Jungar, the latter rising to leadership of the western Mongols in the seventeenth and eighteenth centuries. The Oyrats' Central Eurasian empire has thus come to be known as the Jungar empire. One group of Oyrats who settled nearer Russia were known there as the Kalmuks, a name sometimes applied to the whole group of western Mongols. For further details, see the works of Sechin Jagchid and James Millward.

9. Su Beihai writes that Ablai's mother remarried and that his stepfather was Uyghur. Su, 320.

10. The legend is that he used his father's name, Ablay, as a battle cry, calling out the name as he entered into battle with the Oyrats. Abul Mambet therefore declared that the young warrior, Abul Mansur, would be known by that name. Su, 321.

11. Olcott asserts they were corulers for two decades. Olcott, 40.

12. Many sources say he was khan only after 1771. See Soviet and Japanese sources cited in the bibliography and in Olcott.

13. On the grand council's communication with Ablai, see Millward, 23.

14. Li Sheng, ed., *Xinjiang dui Su (E) maoyi shi, 1600–1990* (1993), 32.

15. For discussion, see Millward, 33.

16. On Zhaohui's career, see Arthur Hummel, *Eminent Chinese of the Ch'ing Period* (1970) 72–74.

17. Li, 32.

18. Millward, 46.

19. Su asserts that Ablai was the great khan, ruling over all three *Juz* (Hordes) beginning in 1744, the year in which the khan of the Small Horde, Abul Haiyur, left for Turkestan. Su, 322.

20. Olcott, 44.

21. Olcott, 67.

22. Godfrey E.P. Hertslet, *Treaties etc. between Great Britain and China; and between China and Foreign Powers; and Orders in Council, Rules, Regulations, Acts of Parliament, Decrees etc. Affecting British Interests in China,* vol. 1 (London: 1908), 475.

23. N.M. Przeval'ski [Przhevalski], *Iz "Zajsana cerez" Xami v "Tibet" i na verxov'ja Zeltoj reki* (From Zaysana through Hami into Tibet and Headwaters of the Yellow River). (St. Petersburg: 1883), 20–21.

24. See further discussion in chapter 5 of the history of Barkol. Sources include *Balikun-Hasake zizhixian gaikuang* (A survey of the Barkol-Kazak Autonomous County) (Urumqi: 1984), 45, and *Mulei-Hasake Zizhixian gaikuang* (A survey of the Mori-Kazak Autonomous County) (Urumqi: 1984), 17–18. On Russian settlements, see George J. Demko, *The Russian Colonization of Kazakhstan, 1866–1917* (1969).

25. See for instance the comments in Olcott, 18–19, and Colin Mackerras, *China's Minority Cultures* (1995), 20–21.

26. Devin DeWeese, *Islamization of Native Religion in the Golden Horde: Baba Tukles and Conversion to Islam in Historical and Epic Tradition* (1994), 9.

27. Eickelman and Piscatori, *Muslim Travellers: Pilgrimage, Migration and Religious Imagination* (1990), 14.

28. Clark also recorded the terms *soyek* and *tap* for these groups. See Milton J. Clark, *Leadership and Political Allocation in Sinkiang Kazak Society* (1955).

29. Halife Altay, *Anayurttan Anadolu'ya* (From my homeland to Anatolia) (1981), 4.

30. Ian Morrison, "Some Notes on the Kazaks of Sinkiang," *Journal of the Royal Central Asian Society* (1948–1949): 69.

31. Hizir Bek Gayretullah *Altaylarda Kanli Gunler* (Bloody days in the Altay) (1977), 107–111; Clark, "Leadership and Political Allocation," 26.

32. Frank Bessac, "Winter at Timurlik 1949–1950," unpublished paper (1991), 23.

33. Lawrence Krader, *Social Organization of the Mongol-Turkic Pastoral Nomads* (1963), 284–285.

34. See examples in "Guanyu Hasakezu de jiehun xisu" (Concerning Kazak marriage customs), *Yili shifan xueyuan xuebao* (Journal of the Ili Teachers' College) (1991): 29–30.

35. Bessac (1991), 11.

36. Ibid., 25.

37. Owen Lattimore, "The Desert Road to Turkestan," *National Geographic Magazine* 55 (1929), 688–689.

Notes to Chapter 3

1. Sun Yatsen, *Memoirs of a Chinese Revolutionary* (1953), 182.

2. Lo, Liang-chien, "Mongolian and Tibetan Affairs," *The Chinese Yearbook* 7 (1946), 271.

3. Ibid. The Ministry of Mongolian and Tibetan Affairs remains a part of the Chinese government on Taiwan.

4. For Xinjiang, see the report of C.C. Ku, "Economic Development of China's Northwest," *China Quarterly* (Shanghai) 4 (1938–1939): 289–297.

5. Chinese Ministry of Information, *China Handbook, 1937–1947* (1947), 341.

6. Han, Lih-wu, "Education," *The Chinese Yearbook* 7 (1946), 787.

7. See Lattimore, *Pivot of Asia,* 79.

8. Ibid., 58, 61.

9. Arthur Hasiotis Jr., *A Study of Soviet Political, Economic, and Military Involvement in Sinkiang from 1928 to 1949,* unpublished Ph.D. dissertation. New York University (1981), 19–20; Demko, *The Russian Colonization of Kazakhstan, 1896–1916* (1969), 78–106.

10. Owen Lattimore, *The Desert Road to Turkestan* (1929), 298–299.

11. Aurel Stein, *Innermost Asia: Detailed Report of Exploration in Central Asia, Kan-su and Eastern Iran,* vol. 2 (London: Oxford University Press, 1928),

553; Douglas Carruthers, *Unknown Mongolia: A Record of Travel and Exploration in North-West Mongolia and Dzungaria* (1814), 360.

12. Richard Yang, "Sinkiang under the Administration of Governor Yang Tsen-hsin, 1911–1928," Central Asiatic Journal 6 (1961), 306–308.

13. Li, 325.

14. Li, 325.

15. Lattimore, *Pivot of Asia,* 66, citing a Russian observer in the region during Jin's governorship.

16. Senior Nationalist army officers traveling in this group were not allowed to enter Xinjiang, according to a recent PRC article. See Yu Rongchun, "Political Role of the Anti-Japanese Volunteer Army in Xinjiang," *Xiyu yanjiu* (Western Regions Studies) 4.15 (December 1993): 21–28. This article asserts that three Han Chinese staged the 1933 coup against Jin, supported by Papingut's Russian troops. Lattimore, however, writes that Papingut and his men mutinied, an account confirmed in Aitchen Wu. See Lattimore, *Pivot of Asia,* 67, and Aitchen K. Wu, *Turkestan Tumult* (1940), 100–115, which does not mention any Chinese in leadership roles of the coup.

17. For a detailed discussion of this event and for information on one of the important Uyghur participants, see L. Benson, "The Life of Yolbars Khan (1888–1971): Pauper, Prince and Politician in Republican Xinjiang," *Opuscula Altaica* (1995), 126–147.

18. For detailed discussion of Sheng and his policies, see Lattimore, *Pivot of Asia,* and Allen Whiting, *Sinkiang: Pawn or Pivot* (1958).

19. Aitchen K. Wu, "The Fourteen Peoples of Chinese Turkistan," *Journal of the West China Border Research Society* 15, series A (1944), 83–93.

20. Lattimore, *Pivot of Asia,* 73

21. It should also be noted that a single issue of a newspaper could reach an extremely wide readership. Copies of newspapers have been traditionally posted on signboards for everyone to read—a practice that continues today. While some people obviously purchased their own copy, many others could have the benefit of the paper without having to buy it. However, it should also be added that newspapers have been used for all manner of things in Xinjiang other than for reading. Up through the early 1980s, for instance, newspaper was still the major source for cigarette paper; it was also used to line shoes. Walter Graham, the British consul at Urumqi in the 1940s, explained that newspaper was used for wrapping all manner of things and was highly desired for that purpose as well as for insulation in house walls. Thus the number of issues a paper sold did not necessarily reflect the public's desire to be informed nor a belief that the news in the paper was factual. Interview with Walter Graham, in England, 1984. L. Benson.

22. U.S. Department of State, Report 751 (June 25, 1942), 38, citing Xinjiang provincial government statistics.

23. See Chang Chih-yi, "Land Utilization and Settlement Possibilities in Sinkiang," *The Geographical Review* 39 (1949): 66.

24. Lattimore, *Pivot of Asia,* 174–175.

25. Li, 409, 554.

26. Lattimore, *Pivot of Asia,* 179.

27. Gayretullah, *Altaylarda Kanli Günler,* 85.

28. Gayretullah, 85–101.

29. Zhang Dajun, *Xinjiang fengbao qishinian* (Xinjiang's seventy turbulent years) (1980), 4215.

30. By the 1940s, phrases such as "the savage Chinese" and the "Chinese oppressor" were common in nationalistic writings of the period. See translations by the U.S. consulate at Urumqi of rebel pamphlets in Linda Benson, *The Ili Rebellion: The Moslem Challenge to Chinese Authority in Xinjiang, 1944–1949* (1990), appendices.

31. On Boke Batur, see Altay, *Anayurttann Anadolu'ya,* 265.

32. Godfrey Lias, *Kazak Exodus* (1956): 35.

33. Ibid., 89.

34. Hasan Oraltay, *Kazak Turkleri* (The Kazak Turks) (1961): 70.

35. This practice was well known to the Kazaks, and had been used for centuries in Central Eurasia as a way of guaranteeing that an agreement would be kept. But for Sheng, it was not so much an adoption of Kazak practice as it was typical of his tactics to ensure compliance with his orders.

36. Whiting, 66–68.

37. Ibid., 67.

38. Oraltay, 76.

39. A. Doak Barnett, *China on the Eve of Communist Takeover* (1963), 275; Zhang, *Xinjiang fengbao qishinian,* 8: 5188.

40. Zhang, *Xinjiang fengbao qishinian,* 8: 5188; Barnett, 275. Although Kazak sources are silent on the issue of whether Osman signed such an agreement with the pro-Soviet Mongols, two Kazak authors write that when Osman was at Tayingol, Mongolia, no less a personage than Choibalsan, leader of the Mongolian government in Ulan Batur, visited Osman at his camp in order to negotiate an arms deal. See Lias, 57–58, and Gayretullah, 91. Burhan, in his memoirs, tells us that the Mongol representative sent to Osman was a man called Mohuaxi, who, along with several others, began arms negotiations with Osman. Baoerhan (Burhan Shahidi) *Xinjiang wushi nian* (Fifty Years in Xinjiang) (1984), 312–313.

41. For discussion of the CCP role in Xinjiang prior to 1949, see Linda Benson, "Chinese Communist Party Contacts with the East Turkestani Movement in Xinjiang, 1944–1950," *Central and Inner Asian Studies* (1992): 1–15.

42. Burhan, 313.

43. The Soviet view of these events is presented in full in the British consular files in London. See British India Office records, L/P&S/12/2359 Col. 12/24 (4), confidential report of April 7, 1944, by British consul, Urumqi, entitled, "Sino-Soviet Relations: Sinkiang-Outer Mongolia Frontier Incidents."

44. For the official Chinese view of the 1944 incident, see *China Yearbook* (Taibei: 1954), 604.

45. *Xinjiang ribao* (March 16, 1944), 1.

46. Jack Chen, *The Sinkiang Story* (1977), 209.

47. Rumors suggested that General Sheng made a sizable contribution, in gold, to the GMD upon his arrival in the national capital in 1944, thereby assuring himself of a safe transition back into the party fold.

48. *Xinjiang ribao* (March 31, 1944), 3.

49. British India Office records, L/P&S/12/2405 Coll. 12/62, "Summary for July," by British Consul Turral, Urumqi, August 2, 1944.

50. Gayretullah, 91–92.

51. British India Office records, L/P&S/12/2405, "Summary for October 1944," British Consul Turral, Urumqi, November 18, 1944.

52. Ibid.

53. Zhang, *Xinjiang fengbao qishinian,* 12: 6348.

54. *Xinjiang ribao* (January 12, 1945), 3.

55. *Xinjiang ribao* (January 12, 1945), 3; Zhang, *Xinjiang fengbao qishinian,* 12: 6356.

56. Gayretullah, 93.

57. Zhang, *Xinjiang fengbao qishinian,* 12: 6350.

58. Ibid.

59. Chinese, Russian, and Kazak sources differ on the date of Chenghua's fall and on the number of troops involved in the fighting. For the Chinese account, see Zhang, *Xinjiang fengbao qishinian,* 12: 6350. For a Russian account, see M. Kutlukov, "The Democratic Movement of the People of South Sinkiang (Kashgaria) between 1945–1947," *Scientific Works and Information* 1 (Tashkent, 1960), 108, citing *Azad Sarqi-Turkestan* of September 5, 1945 and October 10, 1945. The latter is a newspaper that was the official voice of the East Turkestan Republic, the title translating as "Free East Turkestan." A Kazak view is given in Oraltay, 440.

60. Zhang, *Xinjiang fengbao qishinian,* 12: 7306.

61. Ibid., 12: 7307.

62. Morrison, 67–71.

63. The members of the various election committees are listed in *Xinjiang ribao* (September 17, 1946), 3.

64. British Public Record Office, FO 371–53666 (1946), China file 324, reference F 14746, Walter Graham, Urumqi, August 3, 1946.

65. *Xinjiang ribao* (May 11, 1947), 3.

66. British India Office records, L/P&S/12/2360, British Consul Walter Graham's report of February 18, 1947, citing General Song Xilian on the number of troops.

67. Burhan Shahidi (Baoerhan), *Xinjiang Wushi Nian* [Fifty Years in Xinjiang] (1984), 313; Kutlukov, 9.

68. For attacks on Osman, see *Minzhu bao* (Yining), May 19, 1947, 3.

69. Osman himself later reported that he had been defeated by 3,000 Soviet troops, a version of events that remains uncorroborated. See *Xinjiang ribao* (December 23, 1947), 3.

70. *Xinjiang ribao* (December 23, 1947), 2.

71. L. Benson interview with Frank Bessac, Montana, 1981.

72. *Xinjiang-Weiwuer zizhiqu gaikuang* (A survey of the Xinjiang-Uyghur Autonomous Region) (1985), 37–39.

Notes to Chapter 4

1. See Christopher Atwood, "The Japanese Roots of Communist Autonomy Policy in Inner Mongolia," paper presented at the Association of Asian Studies annual meeting, Washington, D.C., 1995, for discussion of CCP activity and Japanese involvement in Inner Mongolia. Clearly, the party's policy drew on the Japanese experience in Manchuria (1931–1945) and on the ambitions of local

Mongol leaders like Ulanhu (Yun Ze), leading to the Foundation of the Inner Mongolian Autonomous Region in May 1947.

2. This program is described briefly in Gutorm Gjessing, "Chinese Anthropology and New China's Policy toward her Minorities," *Acta Sociologica* 2 (1957): 52–53. Translation of relevant parts of the Common Program may be found in Henry G. Schwarz, *Chinese Politics towards Minorities: An Essay and Documents* (1971). See also general discussion of minority policy in works such as Heberer's *China and Its National Minorities: Autonomy or Assimilation?* (1989).

3. A similar program of "self-government" for local areas in China had already been outlined by the Guomindang, which had considered such a system of relative local autonomy to be an important element in fostering national consciousness throughout China.

4. For further details, see Linda Benson, "Liberating Xinjiang from the Rhetoric of Peaceful Liberation," paper presented at the Association of Asian Studies annual meeting, Washington, D.C., 1995.

5. *The Constitution of the People's Republic of China,* art. 68, sec. 5. (Beijing: 1954).

6. *The Constitution of the People's Republic of China* (Beijing: 1986). Emphasis added.

7. Ibid., art. 113, sec. 6, "The Organs of Self-Government of National Autonomous Areas."

8. Ibid.

9. *Minzu tuanjie* (Minority unity), (February 6, 1967), trans. in SCMM, 316, 31.

10. Liu Chun, "Guanyu 'minzu tonghua' wenti," (Regarding the issue of "minority assimilation"), in Central Nationalities Institute Editorial Committee, *Minzu lilun he minzu zhengce, 1951–1983* [Selected theses on nationalities theory and nationalities policy] (1986), 154–160.

11. K. F. Kotov, *Mestnaia natsional'naia avtonomiia v Kitaiskoi Narodnoi Respubliki (na primere Sin'tszian-Uigurskoi avtonomnoi oblasti)* [Autonomy of local nationalities in the People's Republic of China (the Xinjiang-Uyghur Autonomous Region)] (1959), 93

12. American OSS agents were working in Tibet, Xinjiang and Qinghai in 1949–1950, but they were ineffectual. One of the last agents to leave was Frank Bessac, whose works are included in the bibliography. Also see Leonard Clark, *The Marching Wind* (1955).

13. Some of the weapons used by the East Turkestani military were on display in the Xinjiang Regional Museum in Urumqi in 1991, along with other items used by the republic's military in their struggle.

14. The only lengthy account is a book by Sultanov Zayir, a former member of the East Turkestani army. His book includes details such as names of commanders, their new postings after 1949, and the disposition of some units. See Caodanuofu Zayier (Sultanov Zayir), *Wujun de geming licheng* (The revolutionary course of the Fifth Army) (1989).

15. See the useful discussion of this process provided in Harrell, 3–36.

16. That this animosity could also have racial overtones has *never* been acknowledged in official discourse. Nonetheless, recent developments in the region suggest that race is a major factor in ethnic tension. For further discussion, see chapters 6 and 7.

17. Interviews with Uyghurs now resident in the United States uniformly reveal Uyghur disgust with Wang Zhen and his successor, Wang Enmao. An émigré community could be expected to have such a strongly negative assessment of someone in either Wang's position, but it is interesting that not all Chinese officers and officials are regarded in this way. Some, for example, are described as having just done their job, and a few are the butt of jokes for their incompetence. The greatest animosity is invariably reserved for the two Wangs and their shattering impact on the oasis society of southern Xinjiang. When the local population is eventually free to write its own history of those years, the chapters on the two Wangs should be particularly informative on issues such as race and religious policy, the Uyghur perception of what policies were being followed, and the two Wang's motivations for enforcing them in the way that they did.

18. *Renmin ribao* (May 30, 1957), trans. in SCMP, 1551, 28. A refugee from Xinjiang interviewed in Taiwan in the 1980s said that in the middle of the 1950s several meetings were held by minorities, who repeatedly asked Saifudin to attend and answer questions about when real autonomy for Xinjiang would begin. Saifudin refused to attend. Our informant was arrested after speaking out at such a meeting in 1956, before the Hundred Flowers campaign began. He was sentenced to a term of *laogai*—in a labor camp prison—through which he suffered until he was able to escape to Afghanistan in 1968. He ultimately fled to Pakistan and, from there, was assisted to go to Saudi Arabia, where he now lives.

19. Ibid.

20. *Xinjiang ribao* (November 13, 1957), trans. in SCMP 1698, 16.

21. NCNA (New China News Agency) Urumqi (November 30, 1957), trans. in SCMP 1672, 67.

22. Furen Xia, "Marxism vs. Nationalism in Xinjiang: A Major Debate," *Guangming ribao* (April 10, 1958), trans. in SCMP 1764, 26.

23. For an example of an article welcoming such new settlers, see Zhang Shencai, "Let Young People Who Come to Aid and Support Socialist Construction Develop Greater Strength in the Autonomous Region," *Xinjiang ribao* (July 28, 1959), trans. in SCMP, 2120, 15.

24. Figures are mentioned in Zuya and Zhouzutuerti, "Unite and Defend the Socialist Motherland," *Renmin ribao* (September 21, 1969, trans. in SCMP 4508, 9–10. See also June Teufel Dryer, "The Kazakhs of China," 141–177, ed. A. Suhrke and L. Noble, *Ethnic Conflicts in International Relations* (1977), and also her article "Ethnic Minorities in the Sino-Soviet Dispute," in *Soviet Asian Ethnic Frontiers,* ed. W.J. McCagg and Brian Silver, (1979), 195–226. Also see discussion later in this chapter.

25. See for example, NCNA (April 23, 1964), trans. in SCMP 3207, 15.

26. Saifudin (Seyfettin Azizi) was the third minority representative to be the head of the government in Xinjiang since 1912. The first was Mesut Sabri, appointed by the GMD in 1947 (and subsequently executed by the CCP in 1950). The second was Burhan Shahidi who served both the GMD and CCP until 1955. Like his predecessors, Saifudin had experience in dealing with the Chinese, but also like earlier appointees, he owed his position to Han Chinese power. During his first period of service in Xinjiang, he was often called away to Beijing on business, which curtailed his actual influence in the autonomous region, as was perhaps intended.

27. *Xinjiang ribao* (September 7, 1955). A catty equals 0.604 kilograms.

28. NCNA (September 30, 1965), trans. in *CB* 775, 11.

29. Husayin Abaydulla, "The New Sinkiang," *China Reconstructs* 1 (January 1966): 26–30.

30. "State Help Speeds Up Socialist Construction in Sinkiang," *Xinhua Weekly* (October 6, 1975), 19.

31. Robert M. Field, Nicholas Lardy, and Johan Emerson, "A Reconstruction of the Gross Value of Industrial Output by Province in the People's Republic of China 1949–1973," *Foreign Economic Reports, U.S. Department of Commerce* 7 (Washington, D.C.: GPO, 1975).

32. *Renmin ribao* (September 30, 1965), trans. in *CB* 775, 31.

33. See details in "A Brief Account of the Main Organization in Sinkiang Region," *Tianshan fenghuo* (Tianshan Beacon-Fire) (January 15, 1968), trans. in *CB* 855, 1–9.

34. Ibid.

35. "Collection of Documents Concerning the Great Proletarian Cultural Revolution," vol. 1 (May 1967), trans. in *CB* 852, 56.

36. *Tianshan fenghuo* (Tianshan Beacon-Fire) 4–5 (January 15, 1968), trans. in *CB* 852, 56.

37. *Hongqi tongxun* (Red Flag Newsletter) 14 (May 26, 1968), trans. in SCMP 4201, 16.

38. Erkin Alptekin, "Eastern Turkestan: An Overview," *Journal of the Institute of Muslim Minority Affairs* 6.1 (1985): 130.

39. Between 1955 and 1960 there were seven pilgrimages, or *hajj*, to Mecca from Xinjiang, led by China's Islamic Association. Oskar Weggel, *Sinkiang/Xinjiang: Das Zentralasiatische China* [Xinjiang: China's Central Asia] (1984), 197.

40. Institute for Strategic Studies. *Strategic Survey* (1969), 71. See the map on page 272 for further clarification.

41. "Sinkiang Is Advancing in Struggle to Combat and Prevent Revisionism," *Xinhua Weekly* 40 (October 6, 1975), 6.

42. *Xinjiang-Weiwuer zizhiqu gaikuang* (1985), 311–316.

43. "Nationality Policy in China," *Central Asian Survey* 3.1 (1983): 136, citing the vice-director of the Department of Minority Affairs in Urumqi.

44. The 1950 figure is from SCMP 1689, 115; the 1965 figure is from *CB* 775, 30.

45. "Great Victory for Party's Policy of Regional National Autonomy in Sinkiang," *Xinhua Weekly* (October 1, 1975), 35.

46. *Balikun Hasake zizhixian gaikuang* (A survey of the Barkol-Kazak Autonomous County) (1984), 149–150.

47. FBIS-CHI–90–080 (April 25, 1990), 72.

48. JPRS-CPS–85–027 (March 18, 1985), 114.

49. JPRS-CPS–85–031 (April 1, 1985).

50. *Xinjiang-Weiwuer zizhiqu gaikuang* (1985), 39.

51. For an interesting if incomplete account, see George Moseley, *A Sino-Soviet Cultural Frontier: The Ili Kazakh Autonomous Chou* (1966), 28–29.

52. *Xinjiang-Weiwuer zizhiqu gaikuang,* 37.

53. Ibid. 46.

54. Chinese sources use the term *pastoralist*—without indicating whether the people under discussion are Mongol, Tajik, Kirghiz, or Kazak—to name several

of the pastoral peoples of the area. When the term is used in the following discussion, it is because there are no specific statistics for the Kazaks alone.

55. *Xinjiang-Weiwuer zizhiqu gaikuang,* 39.

56. Benson interview with an Uyghur refugee from the Ili Valley, January 1983, Taipei, Taiwan.

57. Ibid.

58. K.F. Kotov, 168.

59. As always, figures dating from this period in China must be used with caution. These are taken from *Xinjiang-Weiwuer zizhiqu gaikuang,* 41.

60. "The New Life of Xinjiang," *Central Asian Review* 4.1 (1956): 74.

61. Audrey Donnithorne, *China's Economic System* (1967), 67.

62. *Xinjiang-Weiwuer zizhiqu gaikuang,* 38–39.

63. Kotov, 117.

64. *Mulei Hasake zizhixian gaikuang* (A survey of Mori-Kazak Autonomous County) (1984), 51.

65. Saifudin, in *Renmin ribao* (October 25, 1959), trans. in SCMP, 2140, 28.

66. *Xinjiang ribao* (January 31, 1959), trans. in SCMP, 2108, 11.

67. *Renmin ribao* (October 10, 1965), trans. in SCMP, 3565, 20. One mu = .0667 hectares.

68. "A Survey of Xinjiang Economic Development," pamphlet in the series *Xinjiang Today,* (1985), 10–11.

69. *Renmin ribao* (June 27, 1958), trans. in *CB* 512, 30.

70. Merhat Sharipzhan, "Kazakhs of Eastern Turkestan in Threshold of 21 [sic] Century," *Bitig: Journal of the Turkish World* (January 1997), 20.

71. "Nationality Policy in Xinjiang, *Central Asian Survey* 3.1 (1983): 136.

72. *Yili Hasake zizhizhou gaikuang* (1985), 84.

73. Ibid., 84.

74. Ibid., 63.

75. *Xinjiang nianjian 1996* (Xinjiang yearbook for 1996), 398.

76. See JoAnna Waley-Cohen, *Exile in Mid-Qing China: Banishment to Xinjiang, 1758–1820* (1991).

77. *Xinjiang nianjian 1995,* 399.

78. FBIS-CHI 88–206 (October 25, 1988), 43.

79. FBIS-CHI–95–188 (September 28, 1995), 86.

80. FBIS-CHI–96–060 (March 27, 1996), 77.

Notes to Chapter 5

1. *Xinjiang nianjian 1995,* 398–399. Numbers are as given in the original source. Figures for minorities add up to 1,979,000 rather than the 1,976,000 given in the source.

2. *Xinjiang nianjian 1992,* 283).

3. On 1950 praise for the East Turkestan Republic, see "Commander Ishak Beg's Revolutionary Struggle," *Xinjiang ribao* (August 29, 1950), 4. Recent praise of the republic appeared in Saifudin's *Tianshan xiongying* (Great eagle of the Tian Shan) (Urumqi: 1988). Additional biographic information on the republic's leaders appeared in *Xinjiang sanqu geming* (Xinjiang's Three Districts

Revolution), by the Xinjiang Three Districts editorial board (Urumqi: 1994).

4. *Yili-Hasake zizhizhou gaikuang* (A survey of the Ili-Kazak Autonomous Prefecture) (1985), 51–52.

5. Ibid., 51.

6. For an account of how the East Turkestan Republic's minzujun transformed into the Fifth Army, see Sultanov Zayir (Caodanuofu Zhayier) *Wujun de geming licheng* (The revolutionary course of the Fifth Army) (1989); for discussion, see Benson, "Liberating Xinjiang."

7. *Yili Hasake zizhizhou gaikuang* (1985), 76. As with the term pastoralists, Chinese sources often refer not to Kazaks but to "herders" as a single category, leaving open the issue of what minorities are under discussion. As Kazaks have constituted the overwhelming majority of herders in the Ili area, the authors here consider the terms *herder* and *Kazak* to be virtually synonymous during the 1950s. After the formation of state farms and ranches, the figures become more problematic as it is not clear from Chinese sources whether the mainly Han Chinese work units of the PCC were also being counted among the herder population. For the small number of other herding populations in Ili, see population figures for Mongols, Kirghiz, and Tajiks given in chapter 1.

8. *Xinjiang ribao* (November 13, 1957), trans. in SCMP 1698, 16.

9. *Guangming ribao* (September 11, 1958), trans. in SCMP 2108, 11.

10. *Xinjiang ribao* (January 31, 1959), trans. in SCMP 2108, 11.

11. For Zhou Enlai's speech, see SCMP 3370, 12.

12. See the account by Zuya and Zhouzutuerti, "Unite and Defend the Socialist Motherland," in *Renmin ribao* (September 21, 1969), trans. in SCMP 4509, 9–10.

13. For example, see the one-sentence report on this in *Yili Hasake zizhizhou gaikuang* (A survey of the Ili-Kazak Autonomous Prefecture) (1985), 198.

14. The fullest account of this is given in Nathan Light, *Qazaqs in the People's Republic of China: The Local Processes of History* (Bloomington: Indiana University, 1994), 72–81.

15. Uyghur informant, personal communication to L. Benson, 1996.

16. *Current Digest of the Soviet Press* (December 30, 1964), 12. Xinjiang also saw a sharp drop in the number of Russians, albeit for different reasons. The Russians numbered 20,000 in 1957 but only 7,245 in 1961. See *China News Analysis*, no. 569 (June 18, 1965), 1–4.

17. Chang Shengcai, "Let Young People Who Come to Aid and Support Socialist Construction Develop Greater Strength in the Autonomous Regions," *Xinjiang ribao* (July 28, 1959), trans. in SCMP 2121, 15, and *Xinjiang ribao* (October 28, 1959), in SCMP 2155, 17.

18. JMJP (People's Daily) (August 9, 1962) in SCMP 2806, 20–22.

19. NCNA (New China News Agency) Urumqi (April 23 1964) in SCMP 3207, 15.

20. Institute for Strategic Studies. *Strategic Survey* (1969), 71.

21. Thomas Hoppe, "Kazak Pastoralism in the Bogda Range," in L. Benson and I. Svanberg, *The Kazaks of China* (1988), 237, citing Bai Huiying, "Qian yi Xinjiang nongcun jinrong gongzuo jingji xiaoyi wenti" (A short discussion of problems in economic efficiency and financial work in Xinjiang Rural Areas), *Xinjiang shehuikexue* (Xinjiang social sciences), 1 (1983), 32.

22. *Xinjiang nianjian 1995*, 398.

23. Hoppe, 210–212.
24. Ibid., 231.
25. Ibid.
26. Ibid., 235.
27. FBIS 90–058 (March 26, 1990), 28–29.
28. FBIS-CHI–95–201 (October 18, 1995), 84.
29. *Xinjiang nianjian 1995,* 398.
30. FBIS-CHI–95–144 (July 27, 1995), 48.
31. FBIS-CHI–90–078 (April 23, 1990), 60–65.
32. FBIS-CHI–88–078 (April 25, 1988), 36.
33. FBIS 90–191 (October 2, 1989).
34. FBIS-CHI 88–215 (November 7, 1988), 67.
35. Statistics from *Chinese Statistical Yearbook 1989,* cited in *Chinese Families in the Post-Mao Era,* ed. Deborah Davis and Stevan Harrell (1993), 3.
36. FBIS-CHI–95–201 (October 18, 1995), 87.
37. *Xinjiang nianjian 1995,* 399.
38. FBIS-CHI–95–201 (October 18, 1995), 88.
39. *Yili-Hasake zizhizhou gaikuang* (1985), 160.
40. SWB/FE/5843/B11/11 (June 20, 1978).
41. Personal communication, L. Benson, June 1996.
42. *Yili-Hasake zizhizhou gaikuang* (1985), 63.
43. Ibid.
44. FBIS-CHI–90–070 (April 11, 1990), 49.
45. FBIS-CHI–95–145 (July 28, 1995), 52.
46. FBIS-CHI–95–201 (October 18, 1995), 87.
47. For an account of the corps in the 1950s, see Basil Davidson, *Turkestan Alive: New Travels in Chinese Central Asia* (1957).
48. *Jiaotong tuce* (Book of Transport and Communication Maps) (1985).
49. *Xinjiang tongzhi* (Xinjiang Information) (1992).
50. Ibid.
51. Ibid.
52. Ibid.
53. Ibid., 9.
54. A. Doak Barnett, *China's Far West* (1994), 400.
55. *Xinjiang-Weiwuer zizhiqu gaikuang* (1985), 317.
56. *Xinjiang nianjian 1995,* 449.
57. *Xinjiang nianjian 1995,* 451.
58. *Balikun-Hasake zizhixian gaikuang* (A Survey of Barkol-Kazak Autonomous County] (1985), 1.
59. Wang Zengyuan, ed. *Xinjiang China* (1989), 32.
60. Joseph Fletcher, "The Military Challenge: The Northwest" in John Fairbank and Kwang-ching Lu, eds., *Cambridge History of China,* vol. 11. (Cambridge: 1989), 239.
61. *Balikun-Hasake zizhixian gaikuang* (1985), 106.
62. Linda Benson and Ingvar Svanberg, eds. *The Kazaks of China* (1988), 88.
63. *Xinjiang nianjian 1995,* 452.
64. Benson and Svanberg, 102.
65. *Xinjiang nianjian 1995,* 433.

66. Foreign Affairs Office of the People's Government of the Xinjiang-Uyghur Autonomous Region. *Xinjiang: A General Survey* (1989), 209.
67. *Xinjiang nianjian 1995,* 443.
68. As virtually no systematic information is available on these small administrative units (e.g., no figures in the press or in yearbooks on population, income, or ethnic composition), it is not yet possible to provide a discussion of these areas.
69. *Mulei-Hasake zizhixian gaikuang* (1985), 38.
70. *Xinjiang tongzhi* (The general annals of Xinjiang), vol. 24. (Urumqi: 1992), 68–72.
71. *Mulei-Hasake zizhixian gaikuang,* 43.
72. Ibid., 58.
73. *Xinjiang-Weiwuer zizhiqu jiaotong tuce* (Xinjiang-Uyghur Autonomous Region transport and communication maps) (Urumqi: 1985).
74. *Mulei-Hasake zizhixian gaikuang* (1985), 58.
75. Ibid., 4, 39, 45, 51, and 57.
76. Ibid., 77–78.
77. *Mulei-Hasake zizhixian gaikuang* (1985), 80.

Notes to Chapter 6

1. Stories appeared in February and March 1997 in the *New York Times,* the *Washington Post,* and the *Far Eastern Economic Review* among other periodicals.
2. For discussion, see Karl H. Menges, "Die Aralo-kaspische Gruppe," in *Philologiaw Turicae Fundamenta* (Wiesbaden: 1959), 434–488; and Ahmet Temir, "Die norwestliche Gruppe der Turksprachen," in *Handbuch der Orientalistik* (Leiden: 1963), 163–173.
3. For examples of the Cyrillic scripts intended for use in Xinjiang, see "Borderlands of Soviet Central Asia: Sinkiang," *Central Asian Review* 4 (1956): 449. See also Paul B. Henze, "Alphabet Changes in Soviet Central Asia and Communist China," *Journal of the Royal Central Asian Society* 44 (1957): 132. A rather biased account of the reforms is also given in Clyde-Ahmed Winters, "Chinese Language Policy and the Muslim Minorities of Xinjiang," *Asian Profile* 10 (1982): 413–419. A more recent, albeit rather general treatment of education and language issues can be found in Colin MacKerras, *China's Minority Cultures* (New York: St. Martin's Press, 1995).
4. New China News Agency, June 22, 1958, cited in SCMP 1799, 28.
5. *Wenzi gaige* (script reform), no. 2 (February 12, 1966), trans. in *Survey of China Mainland Magazines* 531, 35–41.
6. Merhat Sharipzhan, "Kazakhs of Eastern Turkestan in Threshold of 21 [*sic*] Century," *Bitig: Journal of the Turkish World* (January 1997): 18.
7. We have been unable to learn whether novels by Xinjiang-born Kazak authors such as Qabdesh Zhumadilov are available in Xinjiang, in either official or unofficial forms. Zhumadilov left Xinjiang in the 1962 exodus and is the author of several novels and short stories based on the Kazak experience in China. For discussion of his writing, see Nathan Light, "Kazakhs of the Tarbagatai: Ethno-History through the Novel," in *Poetics of Change/Turkish Studies Association Bulletin,* 91–101.

8. Gilbert Chan Fook-lam, *Sinkiang under Sheng Shih-ts'ai, 1933–1944* A.D., Master's thesis, University of Hong Kong (1965), 166.

9. Authors' 1987 interview with Xibo émigré from the Ili area now living in Taiwan.

10. *Yili-Hasake zizhizhou gaikuang* (Survey of the Ili-Kazak Autonomous Prefecture) (1985), 155.

11. This technical school was reportedly founded by Ahmetjan Kasimi, a key figure in the East Turkestan Republic government. See *Yili Hasake zizhizhou gaikuang* (1985), 155.

12. Ibid.

13. Kao Shi-ping, "Sinkiang," *The Chinese Yearbook* 2 (Shanghai: (1936), 173.

14. *Xinjiang-Weiwuer zizhizhou gaikuang* (1985), 210.

15. *Zhongguo 1982 nian renkou pucha ziliao* (China population data yearbook 1982), 240, cited in Heberer, 48.

16. *Zhongguo renkou tongji nianjian* (China population statistics yearbook 1994), 397

17. FBIS-CHI–89–222 (November 20, 1989), 55.

18. Ibid., 54.

19. FBIS-CHI–90–135 (July 13, 1990), 50.

20. FBIS-CHI–90–169 (August 30,1990), 68.

21. FBIS-CHI–95–201 (October 18, 1995), 85.

22. FBIS-CHI–90–250 (December 28, 1990), 53.

23. *Xinjiang nianjian 1992,* 40.

24. FBIS-CHI–90–080 (April 25, 1990), 71.

25. Ibid.

26. FBIS-CHI–95–201 (October 18, 1995), 84.

27. Sharipzhan, 20.

28. FBIS-CHI–88–191 (October 4, 1988), 61.

29. Ibid. Also see discussion in chapter 5 on income in the Kazak areas of Xinjiang.

30. Ibid.

31. FBIS-CHI–90–080 (April 25, 1990), 71.

32. Heberer, 89.

33. Ibid.

34. FBIS-CHI–88–089 (May 9, 1988), 52.

35. FBIS-CHI–88–183 (September 21, 1988), 64.

36. FBIS-CHI–88–118 (June 20, 1988), 65.

37. Ibid.

38. Ibid.

39. Xu Xifa, *Zhongguo xiaoshu minzu jihua shengyu gailun* (An introduction to China's minority nationalities family planning) (Urumqi: 1995), 23–24. Statistics for 1990 gave a natural population growth rate of between 15 and 25 per thousand in Ili and Altay, but the summary published in *Xinjiang ribao* did not give statistics by minority group. For the *Xinjiang ribao* report, see FBIS-CHI–90–250 (December 28, 1990), 53.

40. Xu Xifa, *Zhongguo xiaoshu minzu jihua shengyu gailun* (An introduction to China's minority nationalities family planning) (1995), 22.

41. FBIS-CHI–90–083 (April 30, 1990), 65.

42. Ibid.

43. FBIS-CHI–88–208 (October 27, 1988), 57.

44. FBIS-CHI–88–227 (November 25, 1988), 62.

45. FBIS-CHI–88–136 (August 22, 1985), 52.

46. FBIS-CHI–88–208 (October 27, 1988), 52, citing the Hong Kong paper *Mingbao.*

47. Ibid.

48. FBIS-CHI–88–227 (November 25, 1988), 66.

49. FBIS-CHI–89–097 (May 22, 1989), 65.

50. FBIS-CHI–89–101 (May 26, 1989), 64.

51. FBIS-CHI–89–116 (June 19, 1989), 69–70.

52. FBIS-CHI–90–080 (April 25, 1990), 65.

53. For details on the Baren incident, see the FBIS-CHI reports for April, May, and June 1990.

54. FBIS-CHI–90–083 (April 30, 1990), 63.

55. Reports on the bus bombings appeared in the *London Times* (March 3, 1992): *The Guardian* (March 9, 1992), and in the Turkestani publication *Eastern Turkestan Information* 12 (March 1992). In 1993, a bomb exploded in a hotel in Kashgar, followed by bombings of factories in Kashgar and Urumqi; bombs also exploded on public buses in Urumqi that June.

56. FBIS-CHI–94–057 (December 22, 1994), 89.

57. *Xinjiang nianjian 1992,* 40–41.

58. JPRS-CAR–94–057 (December 22, 1994), 89.

59. SWB/FE/2336 G/6 (June 22, 1995).

60. "Xinjiang terrorists killed in police battle," *South China Morning Post* (Hong Kong) (May 22, 1996), 1. See also Steve Mufson, "Tibetans, Muslims Clash with Beijing, *Washington Post* (May 31, 1996).

61. *New York Times* article in the *Oakland Press* (March 8, 1997), A10.

Notes to Chapter 7

1. In 1986, the authors were refused permission to visit Sairam Lake, near the Soviet border, although the English-language *China Daily* featured a picture of "foreign visitors" at Sairam that same year. When asked if the story were untrue, officials at Urumqi's Public Security Bureau simply stated that the foreigners were overseas Chinese compatriots from Hong Kong and Taiwan and that the area was not yet open to "other" foreign visitors.

2. I. Svanberg, "Contemporary Changes among the Kazaks," in *Ethnicity, Minorities, and Cultural Encounters*, ed. I. Svanberg (1991), 85. As a participant in an international conference held in Peshawar, Pakistan, in 1992, I was told that the Chinese would not allow any scholar or official to attend the meetings. An international conference sponsored by the School of Oriental Studies, London, planned for 1993, was canceled when the Chinese government without explanation refused to issue the Kazak and Uyghur panelists travel documents. L. Benson.

3. Martha Brill Olcott, *Central Asia's New States* (1996), 62.

4. Ibid.

5. FBIS-CHI–89–163 (August 24, 1989), 2.

6. FBIS-CHI–89–140 (July 24, 1989), 7.

7. FBIS-CHI–95–180 (September 18, 1995), 7.

8. Stanley W. Toops, "Crossing the Border: Xinjiang's Trade and Tourism with Neighboring Countries," paper presented at the Association of Asian Studies Annual Meeting, 1994.

9. Ibid., 15.

10. Ibid., 4.

11. Ibid., figure 8, citing Abulat Abruxit and Han Xuewang, eds., *Duiwai kaifang de Xinjiang kouan* (Externally open ports in Xinjiang) (1993).

12. Liu Weiling, "Border Trade a Boon for Xinjiang," *Beijing Review* (January 23–29, 1995): 5.

13. FBIS-CHI–95–180 (September 18, 1995), 7.

14. ITAR-TASS World Service, Moscow radio broadcast, May 7, 1997.

15. An overview of the contemporary ecocide in Kazakstan, Uzbekistan, Turkmenistan, and Xinjiang is given in M. Andersson and I. Svanberg, *Fran Rio till Aral: om miljomord i Centralasien* (1995).

Bibliography

Abramzon, S. M. "The Kirgiz of the Chinese People's Republic," *Central Asian Review*, Vol. 11 (1963).

Allworth, Edward, ed. *Central Asia: A Century of Russian Rule.* New York: Columbia University Press, 1967; reissued by Duke University Press, 1989.

Alptekin, Erkin. "East Turkestan: An Overview," *Journal of the Institute of Muslim Minority Affairs*, 6:1 (1985).

Alptekin, Isa Yusuf. *Dogu Turkistan Davasi.* [A Petitioner for East Turkestan]. Istanbul: Otag Matbaasi, 1975.

Altay, Halife. "Hur Dunyada Turkistan Muhacirleri," [Never Free: Turkestani Refugees], *Turkeli*, 5 (1978), 16–22.

———. *Anayurttan Anadolu'ya* [From My Homeland to Anatolia]. Istanbul: n.p., 1981.

Andersson, Magnus, and Ingvar Svanberg. *Från Rio till Aral: Om miljömord i Centralasien* [From Rio to Aral: Ecocide in Central Asia]. Stockholm: Brevskolan, 1995.

Anonymous. *China: A Geographical Sketch.* [English edition] Beijing: Foreign Languages Press, 1974.

Anonymous. *Xinjiang: The Land and the People.* [English edition] Beijing: New World Press, 1989.

Atwood, Christopher. "The East Mongolian Revolution and Chinese Communism," *Mongolian Studies*, Vol. XV (1992), 12–83.

Aubin, Françoise. "Chinese Islam: In Pursuit of Its Source," *Central Asian Survey*, 5:2 (1986), 73–80.

Bacon, Elizabeth. *Central Asians Under Russian Rule.* Ithaca, New York: Cornell University Press, 1966.

———. *Obok: A Study of Social Structure in Eurasia.* New York: Viking Fund Publications, 1958.

Bailey, Lt-Col. F.M. *Mission to Tashkent.* London: Jonathan Cape, 1946.

Balzer, Marjorie. *Shamanic Worlds: Rituals and Lore of Siberia and Central Asia.* Armonk, New York: M.E. Sharpe, Inc., 1996.

Baoerhan [Burhan Shahidi]. *Xinjiang wushinian* [Fifty years in Xinjiang]. Urumqi: Historical Materials Press, 1984.

Barkol-Kazak Autonomous County Survey Compilation Committee, *Balikun Ha-*

sake zizhixian gaikuang [A Survey of Barkol-Kazak Autonomous County]. Urumqi, Xinjiang: Xinjiang People's Press, 1984.

Barnett, A. Doak. *China on the Eve of Communist Takeover*. London: Frederick A. Praeger, Inc., 1963.

————. *China's Far West: Four Decades of Change*. Boulder, Colorado: Westview Press, 1993.

Barthold, W. *Turkestan Down to the Mongol Invasion*. London: Luzac and Co. Ltd., 1958.

Bawden, C.R. *The Modern History of Mongolia*. London: Weidenfeld and Nicolson, 1968.

Bayangolin-Mongol Autonomous County Survey Compilation Committee, *Bayanguoleng-Menggu zizhizhou gaikuang* [A survey of Bayangolin-Mongol Autonomous Prefecture]. Urumqi: Xinjiang People's Press, 1985.

Belenitsky, Aleksandr. *Central Asia*. Translated by James Hogarth. London: The Cresset Press, 1969.

Beloff, Max. *Soviet Policy in the Far East 1944-1951*. London: Oxford University Press, 1953.

Bennigsen, Alexandre. "The Bolshevik Conquest of the Moslem Borderlands," in Thomas Hammond, ed. *The Anatomy of Communist Takeovers*. London: Yale University Press, 1975.

Bennigsen, Alexandre, and Marie Broxup. *The Islamic Threat to the Soviet State*. London: Croom Helm, 1983.

Benson, Linda. *The Ili Rebellion: The Moslem Challenge to Chinese Authority in Xinjiang 1944–1949*. Armonk, New York: M.E. Sharpe, Inc., 1990.

————. "Osman Batur: The Kazaks' Golden Legend," in L. Benson and I. Svanberg, eds. *The Kazaks of China: Essays on an Ethnic Minority*. Uppsala, Sweden: Acta Universitatis Upsaliensia, 1988.

————. "Uygur Politicians of the 1940s: Mehmet Emin Bugra, Isa Yusuf Alptekin and Mesut Sabri," *Central Asian Survey* 10:4 (1991), 87–113.

————. "Liberating Xinjiang from the Rhetoric of Liberation," unpublished conference paper presented at the Association of Asian Studies annual meeting, Washington, D.C., 1995.

————. "Contested History: Issues in the Historiography of Inner Asia's Uighurs," *Toronto Studies in Central and Inner Asia*, 2 (1996), 115–131.

Benson, Linda, and Ingvar Svanberg, "The Russians in Xinjiang: From Immigrants to National Minority," *Central Asian Survey*, 8:2 (1989), 97–129.

Benson, Linda, and Ingvar Svanberg, eds. *The Kazaks of China: Essays on an Ethnic Minority*. Uppsala, Sweden: Acta Universitatis Upsaliensis, 1988.

Bessac, Frank. "Culture Types of Northern and Western China." Unpublished Ph.D. dissertation, University of Wisconsin, 1963.

————. "Co-variation between Interethnic Relations and Social Organizations in Inner Asia," *Papers of the Michigan Academy of Science, Arts and Letters*, Vol. 50, 1965.

————. "Cult Unit and Ethnic Unit—Process and Symbolism," in June Helm, ed. *Essays on the Problem of the Tribe: Proceedings of the 1967 Annual Spring Meeting of the American Ethnological Society*. Seattle: University of Washington Press, 1968.

————. "Revolution and Government in Inner Mongolia: 1945-50." *Papers of*

the Michigan Academy of Science, Arts and Letters 1 (1965), 415-429.
————. "Winter at Timurlik 1949–1950." Unpublished paper presented at the Workshop, "The Kazakhs on the Sino-Soviet Frontier: National Identities and the Transformation of Tradition," University of Southern California, Los Angeles, December 14–15, 1990.
Bortala-Mongol Autonomous Prefecture Survey Compilation Committee. *Bolotala-Menggu zizhizhou gaikuang* [A survey of Bortala-Mongol Autonomous Prefecture]. Urumqi, Xinjiang: Xinjiang People's Press, 1985.
Boorman, Howard. L., and Richard C. Howard, eds. *Biographical Dictionary of Republican China.* 2 vols. New York: Columbia University Press, 1967-69.
Broomhall, Marshall. *Islam in China.* London: 1910; reprinted edition, New York: Paragon Book Reprint Corp., 1966.
Brugger, Bill. *China: Liberation and Transformation 1942-62.* London: Croom Helm, 1981.
Bruchi, Michael. "The Effect of the USSR's Language Policy on the National Languages of Its Turkic Population," in Yaacov Ro'i, ed., *The USSR and The Muslim World.* London: George Allen and Unwin, 1984.
Bruk, S. I. "Etnicheskii sostav i razmeshchenie naseleniia v Sin'czianskom Uigurskom avtonomnon raione Kitaiskoi narodnoi respubliki" [Ethnic composition and distribution of the population in the Xinjiang-Uyghur Autonomous Region of the People's Republic of China], *Sovetskaia etnografija,* 1956:2, 89–94.
Brunnert, H.S. and V.V. Hagelstrom. *Present Day Political Organization of China.* Translated by A. Beltchenko and E.E. Moran. Shanghai: Kelly and Walsh, 1912
Cable, Mildred and Francesca French. *The Gobi Desert.* London: Hodder and Stoughton, 1942.
Caodanuofu Zayier. See Zayir, Sultanov.
Carruthers, Douglas. *Unknown Mongolia. A Record of Travel and Exploration in Northwest Mongolia and Dzungaria.* Vol 12. London: n.p., 1914.
Castagne, J. "Les tamgas des Kirgizes (Kazaks)," *Revue du monde Musulman* 39 (1921), 30–64.
Central Nationalities Institute Editorial Committee. *Minzu lilun he minzu zhengce lunwenxian, 1951–1983* [Selected theses on nationalities theory and nationalities policy 1951–1983]. Beijing: Central Nationalities Institute Press, 1986.
Chan, F. Gilbert, ed. *China at the Crossroads: Nationalists and Communists, 1927-1949.* Boulder, Colorado: Westview Press, 1980.
Chan, Fook-lam Gilbert. "Sinkiang Under Sheng Shih-ts'ai." Unpublished Master's thesis, University of Hong Kong, 1965.
Chang Chih-yi. "Land Utilization and Settlement Possibilities in Sinkiang," *The Geographical Review* 39 (1949), 68–74.
Changji-Hui Autonomous Prefecture Survey Compilation Committee. *Changji Huizizhizhou gaikuang* [A general survey of the Changji-Hui Autonomous Prefecture]. Urumqi: Xinjiang People's Press, 1985.
Chen, Jack. *The Sinkiang Story.* London: Collier Macmillan, 1977.
Chen, Yunbin, ed. *Ili-Hasake zizhizhou gaikuang* [A survey of the Ili-Kazak Autonomous Prefecture]. Urumqi, Xinjiang: Xinjiang People's Press, 1985.
Chesneau, Jean, ed. *Popular Movements and Secret Societies in China 1840-1950.* Stanford: Stanford University Press, 1972.

Chiang, Chung-cheng (Chiang Kaishek). *Soviet Russia in China*. New York: Farrar, Straus & Ludahy, 1957.

Chinese Ministry of Information. *China Handbook 1937-43*. New York: The MacMillan Co., 1943.

Chou, Nailene Josephine. "Frontier Studies and Changing Frontier Administration in Late Ch'ing China: The Case of Sinkiang 1759-1911." Unpublished Ph.D. dissertation, University of Washington, 1976.

Clark, Leonard. *The Marching Wind*. London: Hutchinson, 1955.

Clark, Milton J. "How the Kazaks Fled to Freedom," *National Geographic Magazine* 106 (1955), 621–644.

————. *Leadership and Political Allocation in Sinkiang Kazak Society*. Unpublished Ph.D. dissertation, Harvard University, 1955.

Clem, Ralph. "The Frontier and Colonialism in Russian and Soviet Central Asia," in Robert A. Lewis, ed., *Geographic Perspectives on Soviet Central Asia*. London: Routledge, 1992.

Clubb, O. Edmund. *China and Russia: The "Great Game."* London: Columbia University Press, 1971.

Comrie, Bernard. *The World's Major Languages*. New York: Oxford University Press, 1987.

Conquest, Robert. *Soviet Nationalities Policy in Practice*. New York: Frederick Praeger, 1967.

Cressey, George S. *Asia's Land and Peoples*. New York: McGraw-Hill Book Co. Inc., 1951.

Czaplicka, M.A. *The Turks of Central Asia*. London: Curzon Press, 1918.

Dabbs, Jack A. *History of the Discovery and Exploration of Chinese Turkestan*. The Hague, Netherlands: Mouton & Co., 1963.

Davidson, Basil. *Turkestan Alive: New Travels in Chinese Central Asia*. London: Jonathan Cape, 1957.

Davis, Deborah and Stevan Harrell, eds. *Chinese Families in the Post-Mao Era*. Berkeley: University of California Press, 1993.

Demko, George J. *The Russian Colonization of Kazakhstan, 1896–1916*. Bloomington, Indiana: Indiana University Publications, Uralic-Altaic Series, Vol. 99, 1969.

DeWeese, Devin. *Islamization and Native Religion in the Golden Horde: Baba Tukles and Conversion to Islam in Historical and Epic Tradition*. University Park, Pennsylvania: Pennsylvania State University Press, 1994.

Dingelstedt, Viktor. "Le droit coutumier des Kirghiz," *Revue General du Droit, de la Legislation et de la Jurisprudence*. Vol. 14 (1890), 141–155, 213–225, 320–330, 451–462, 516–525.

Dogru, Sirzat. "Buyuk Turkistan Mucahidi, Osman Batur'u Aniyoruz," [Great Turkestan's Resistance Fighter: In Memory of Osman Batur] *Turkeli* 1:1 (1968), 11–14.

Donnithorne, Audrey. *China's Economic System*. London: George Allen and Unwin Ltd., 1967.

Dreyer, June Teufel. *China's Forty Millions*. London: Harvard University Press, 1976.

————. "The Kazakhs in China," in A. Suhrke and L.G. Noble, eds., *Ethnic Conflict and International Relations*. New York: Praeger, 1977, 146–177.

————. "Ethnic Minorities in the Sino-Soviet Dispute," in *Soviet Asian Ethnic Frontiers*, ed. William O. McCagg and Brian D. Silver. New York: Pergamon 1979.

Eastman, Lloyd. *Seeds of Destruction*. Stanford: Stanford University Press, 1984.

Eickelmann, Dale E. and James Piscatori, editors. *Muslim Travellers: Pilgrimages, Migration and Religious Imagination*. Berkeley, California: University of California Press, 1990.

Etherton, P.T. *In the Heart of Asia*. London: Constable and Co. Ltd., 1925.

Ekvall, Robert. *Cultural Relations on the Kansu-Tibetan Border*. Chicago: University of Chicago Press, 1939.

Fei, Hsiao-tung. "Ethnic Identification in China," *Social Sciences in China* 1:1 (1980), 94–107.

Finke, Peter, *Nomadismus der Kasachen in der Westmongolei*. Unpublished thesis, Freie Universität, Berlin, 1995.

Fleming, Peter. *Travels in Tartary*. London: Jonathan Cape, 1948.

Fletcher, Joseph. "Ch'ing Inner Asia c. 1800," in John King Fairbank and K. C. Liu, eds. *The Cambridge History of China*, Vol. 10, Part I. New York: Cambridge University Press, 1980.

————. "The Heyday of the Ch'ing Order in Mongolia, Sinkiang and Tibet," in John King Fairbank and K.C. Liu, eds. *The Cambridge History of China*, Vol. I, Part I. New York: Cambridge University Press, 1980.

————. "The Military Challenge: The Northwest," in John King Fairbank and K.C. Liu, eds. *The Cambridge History of China*, Vol. 11. New York: Cambridge University Press, 1989.

Forde, C. Daryll. "The Kazak: Horse and Sheep Herders of Central Asia," in Y. A. Cohen, comp. *Man in Adaptation: The Cultural Present*. Chicago: Aldine Publishing Co., 1968, 299–309.

Foreign Affairs Office of the People's Government of the Xinjiang-Uighur Autonomous Region, *Xinjiang: A General Survey*. Transl. Zheng Ping and Yang Yaohua. Beijing: New World Press, 1989.

Foster, Charles R. *Nations Without States: Ethnic Minorities in Western Europe*. New York: Praeger Publishers, 1980.

Gansu Province Nationalities Research Institute, ed. *Yisilan Jiao zai Zhongguo* [The Muslim Religion in China]. Gansu: Ningxia People's Press, 1982.

Gayretullah, Hizir Bek. *Altaylarda Kanli Gunler* [Bloody days in the Altay]. Istanbul: Ahmet Sit Matbaasi, 1977.

Geertz, Clifford. *Islam Observed*. New Haven, Connecticut: Yale University Press, 1968.

Geng Shimin. "On the Fusion of Nationalities in the Tarim Basin and the Formation of the Modern Uighur Nationality," *Central Asian Survey* 3:4 (1984), 1–14.

Gjessing, Gutorm. "Chinese Anthropology and New China's Policy toward her Minorities," *Acta Sociologica*, 2 (1957), 45–69.

Gladney, Dru. *Muslim Chinese: Ethnic Nationalism in the People's Republic*. Cambridge, Massachusetts: Harvard University Press, 1991.

Gokalp, Ziya. *The Principles of Turkism*. Translated by Robert Deuereux. Leiden, Netherlands: E.J. Brill, 1968.

Gokturk, Hamit. "Osman Batur Islamoglu," *Dogu Turkistan* 2:8 (1981), 20–21.

Harrell, Stevan, ed. *Cultural Encounters on China's Ethnic Frontiers.* Seattle: University of Washington Press, 1995.

Hasiotis Jr, Arthur. *A Study of Soviet Political, Economic, and Military Involvement in Sinkiang from 1928 to 1949.* Ph.D. dissertation, New York University, 1981.

Hayit, Baymirza. *Soviet Russian Colonialism and Imperialism in Turkestan as an Example of the Soviet Type of Colonialism of an Islamic People in Asia.* Koln: n. p., 1965.

Heberer, Thomas. *China and Its National Minorities: Autonomy or Assimilation.* Armonk, New York: M.E. Sharpe, Inc., 1989.

Hedin, Sven. *The Flight of Big Horse.* Translated by F.H. Lyon. New York: E.P. Dutton and Co., Inc., 1936.

Henze, Paul B. "Alphabet Changes in Soviet Central Asia and Communist China," *Journal of the Royal Central Asian Society,* 4 (1956).

Hertslet. Godfrey E.P. *Treaties etc., between Great Britain and China; and between China and Foreign Powers; and Orders in Council, Rules, Regulations, Acts of Parliament, Decrees, etc. affecting British Interests in China.* London: Harrison and Son, 1908.

Heyd, Uriel. *Foundations of Turkish Nationalism: The Life and Teachings of Ziya Gokalp.* London: Luzac & Co. Ltd., 1950.

Holdsworth, Mary. *Turkestan in the 19th Century.* London: Central Asian Research Centre, in association with St. Anthony's College, Oxford, Soviet Affairs Study Group, 1959.

Hoppe, Thomas. "Observations on Uygur Land Use in Turpan County, Xinjiang—a Preliminary Report on Field Work in Summer 1985," *Central Asiatic Journal* 32:3–4 (1986), 224–251.

———. *Xinjiang: Provisional Bibliography 2.* Wiesbaden: Otto Harrassowitz, 1987.

———. "Kazak Pastoralism in the Bogda Range," in L. Benson and I. Svanberg, eds. *The Kazaks of China: Essays on an Ethnic Minority.* Uppsala, Sweden: Studia Multiethnica Upsaliensia, 1988.

Hostler, Charles Warren. *Turkism and the Soviets.* London: George Allen and Unwin Ltd., 1957.

Hsieh, Jiann. "China's Nationality Policy: Its Development and Problems," *Anthropos* 81 (1986), 1–20.

Hsu, Immanuel C.Y. *The Ili Crisis: A Study of Sino-Russian Diplomacy 1871-1881.* London: Oxford, Clarendon Press, 1965.

Hudson, Alfred E. *Kazak Social Structure.* New Haven, Connecticut: Yale Univesity Press, 1938.

Hummel, Arthur. *Eminent Chinese of the Ch'ing Period.* [reprint] Taipei: Ch'eng Wen Publishing Co., 1970.

Ili-Kazak Autonomous Prefecture survey Compilation Committee. *Yili-Hasake zizhizhou gaikuang* [A survey of the Ili-Kazak Autonomous Prefecture]. Urumqi: Xinjiang People's Press, 1985.

Institute for Strategic Studies. *Survey of Strategic Studies.* London: n.p. 1970.

Islam, Qabisuli. *Kereyler kerweni (tariykhiy monografiyaliq qishwqasi soliw)* [The caravan of the Kereys (a brief historical monograph)]. Istanbul: Olgiy Press, 1978.

Ismail, Mohammed Sa'id and Mohammed Aziz Ismail. *Moslems in the Soviet Union and China.* Transl. US Government Joint Publications Research Service [JPRS] 3936 (1960). Tehran, Iran: Privately printed pamphlet, published as Vol. 1, Hejira 1380 (1960).

Jagchid, Sechin. "The Failure of a Self-determination Movement: The Inner Mongolian Case," in William O. McCagg and Brian D. Silver, eds., *Soviet Asian Ethnic Frontiers.* New York: Pergamon Press, 1979.

Janabil, Jiger. "A Revival of a Tradition: Celebration of Navrez Meram," *Inner Asia Report: Newsletter of the Harvard Students for Inner Asia.* No. 7 (Fall 1990), 9–10.

Jankowiak, William R. *Sex, Death and Hierarchy in a Chinese City: An Anthropological Account.* New York: Columbia University Press, 1993.

Jarring, Gunnar. "Owner's Mark·Among the Turks of Central Asia," *Beitrage zur Turkologie und Zentralasienkunde.* Weisbaden: Veröffentlichungen der Societatis Uralo-Altaica, 1981.

———. "The New Romanized Alphabet for Uighur and Kazakh and Some Observations on the Uighur Dialect of Kashgar," *Central Asiatic Journal* 25:3–4 (1981), 230–244.

———. *On the Distribution of Turk Tribes in Afghanistan.* Lund, Sweden: Lunds Universtitets Arsskrift, 1939.

———. "Some Notes on Central Asian Turkic Place Names," *Bulletin of the Geological Institution of Uppsala.* 40 (1961), 467–478.

———. *Return to Kashgar.* Transl. Eva Claeson. Durham, North Carolina: Duke University Press, 1986.

———. "The Toponym Takla-makan," *Turkic Languages,* 1:2 (1997), 227–241.

Kaluzynski, Stanislaw. *Die Sprache des Mandschurischen Stammes Sibe aus der Gegend von Kuldscha.* Vol 1. Warszawa: Panstwowe Wydawn Naukowe, 1977.

Kamberi, Dolkun. *The Study of Medieval Uyghur Drama and Related Cultural Phenomena.* Unpublished Ph.D. dissertation, Columbia University, 1995.

Kao, Shi-ping. "Sinkiang," *The China Yearbook 1936–37.* Shanghai: The North China Daily News and Herald, Ltd., 1937.

Kara, Abdulvahap. "Baslarken," *Avrupa Kazak Turkleri Bulteni* 1:1 (Spring 1993), 1.

Karutz, Richard. "Von kirgisischer Hochzeit und Ehe auf Mangyschlag," *Globus* 10 (1919), 37–42.

———. *Unter Kirgisen und Turkmenen. Aus dem Leben der Steppe.* Leipzig: Klinkhardt & Biermann, 1911.

Kazak, Fuad. *Ost-Turkistan zwischen den Grossmächten: Beitrag zur wirtschaftskunde Osttürkistans.* Berlin: Ost-Europa Verlag, 1937.

Kedourie, Elie, ed. *Nationalism in Asia and Africa.* London: Weidenfeld and Nicolson, 1971.

Khazanov, Anatoly M. *Nomads and the Outside World.* Madison, Wisconsin: University of Wisconsin Press, 1994.

Klein, Donald W., and Anne B. Clark. *Biographic Dictionary of Chinese Communism 1921–1965.* Cambridge, Massachusetts: Harvard University Press, 1971.

Kotov, Konstantin F. *Mestnaia natsional'naia avtonomiia v Kitaiskoi Narodnoi Respubliki (na primere Sin'tszian-Uigurskoi avtonomnoi oblasti)* [Autonomy of local nationalities in the Chinese People's Republic (the Xinjiang-Uyghur

Autonomous Region)]. Moscow: gos. Izd-vo iurid. litry, 1959.

Krader, Lawrence. *Peoples of Central Asia*. Bloomington, Indiana: Indiana University Press, 1963.

———. "Ethnonym of Kazakh," in Nickolai Poppe, ed. *American Studies in Altaic Linguistics*. Bloomington, Indiana: Indiana University Press, 1962.

———. and Ivor Wayne. *The Kazakhs: A Background Study for Psychological Warfare*. Washington, D.C.: Human Resources Research Office Technical Report, 1955.

———. "Principles and Structures in the Organization of the Asiatic Steppe Pastoralists," *Southwestern Journal of Anthropology*. 12:2 (1955), 67–92.

———. *Social Organization of the Mongol-Turkic Pastoral Nomads*. The Hague, Netherlands: Mouton & Co., 1963.

Ku, C. C. "Economic Development of China's Northwest," *China Quarterly* (Shanghai) No. 4 (1938–1939), 289–297.

Kuropatkin, A.N. *Kashgaria: Historical and Geological Sketch of the Country, Its Military Strength, Industries and Trade*. Translated by Major W.E. Gowan. Calcutta: Thacker, Spink & Co., 1882.

Kutlukov, M. "The National Liberation Movement of 1944–1949 in Xinjiang as Part of the Chinese People's Revolution," in *Collected Works of the Graduate School of Social Science*. Vol. 1. Tashkent: Uzbek SSR Academy of Science, 1958, 255–271.

———. "The Democratic Movement of the People of South Xinjiang (Kashgaria) Between 1945–1947," *Scientific Works and Information* 1. Tashkent: Department of Social Sciences, Academy of Science, Uzbek SSR, 1960.

Lamb, Alastair. *Asian Frontiers*. London: Pall Mall Press, 1968.

Lattimore, Owen and Eleanor. "Mongolia, Sinkiang and Tibet," in Lawrence Rosinger, ed. *The State of Asia*. New York: Alfred Knopf, 1951.

———. *Pivot of Asia*. Boston: Little, Brown and Co., 1950.

———. *Nationalism and Revolution in Mongolia*. New York: Oxford University Press, 1955.

———. *Studies in Frontier History*. London: Oxford University Press, 1962.

———. *High Tartary*. Boston: Little, Brown & Co., 1930.

———. *The Desert Road to Turkestan*. Boston: Little, Brown & Co., 1929.

Le Coq, Albert von. *Buried Treasures of Chinese Turkestan*. Translated by Anna Barwell. London: George Allen & Unwin Ltd., 1926.

Levshin, Aleksis [de Levchine, Alexis]. *Déscription des hordes et des steppes Kirghiz-Kazaks ou Kirghiz-Kaissaks*. Paris: Imprimerie royale, 1840.

Li, Donghui, ed. *China Western Border Trade*. Urumqi, Xinjiang: Art and Photography Publishing, 1993.

Li, Jinwei. *Xinjiang fengyun* [Xinjiang storm clouds]. Hong Kong: Haiwai Shudian, 1947.

Li, Jinwei, and Shui Jiantong, eds. *Xinjjiang wenti*. [The Xinjiang Problem]. Hong Kong: Haiwai Shudian, 1947.

Li, Sheng. *Xinjiang dui Su (E) Maoyishi 1600–1990*. [Xinjiang's Trade with the Soviet Union (Russia) from 1600–1990]. Urumqi, Xinjiang: Xinjiang People's Press, 1993.

Lias, Godfrey. *Kazak Exodus*. London: Evans Brothers Limited, 1956.

Liu, Guanghong, ed. *Zhongguo minzu gongju wenxian cidian* [China's Nationalities Reference Document Dictionary]. Beijing: Reform Press, 1995.

Light, Nathan. *Qazaqs in the People's Republic of China: The Local Processes of History.* Occasional Paper No. 22. Bloomington, Indiana: MacArthur Scholars Series, 1994.

————. "Kazakhs of the Tarbagatai: Ethno-History through the Novel," *Turkish Studies Association Bulletin*, 17:2 (1992), 91–101.

Lipman, Jonathan. "Ethnicity and Politics in Republican China; The Ma Family Warlords of Gansu," *Modern China* 10:3 (1984), 285–316.

————. "Ethnic Violence: Hans and Huis on the Northwestern Frontier," in Jonathan Lipman and Stevan Harrell, eds. *Violence in China: Essays in Culture and Counter-Culture.* Albany, New York: State University of New York Press, 1990.

Ma, Jiangsheng, Cheng Suoluo, and Mu Guangwen, eds. *Weiwuer shiliao jianbian* [Concise edition of historical materials on the Uyghurs]. Vol. 1, 2. Beijing: People's Press, 1981.

McCagg, William O., and Brian D. Silver, eds. *Soviet Asian Ethnic Frontiers.* New York: Pergamon Press, 1979.

Mackerras, Colin. *The Uighur Empire (744-840).* Canberra: Centre of Oriental Studies, the Australian National University, 1968.

————. *China's Minority Cultures.* New York: St. Martin's Press, 1995.

Maenchen-Helfen, Otto. *The World of the Huns.* Berkeley: University of California Press, 1973.

Manjani, Niqmet [Nikmet Menjani]. "The Spread of Islam Among the Kazak People," in *The Legacy of Islam in China.* Unpublished conference papers from the Harvard University International Symposium in Memory of Joseph F. Fletcher, 1989, 733–783.

Mannerheim, C. G. E. *Across Asia from West to East in 1906–1908.* Helsinki: Suomalais-Urgrilainen Seura, 1940.

Marshall, Richard H. Jr. *Aspects of Religion in the Soviet Union 1917-1967.* Chicago: University of Chicago Press, 1971.

Massell, Gergory J. *The Surrogate Proletariat: Moslem Women and Revolutionary Strategies in Soviet Central Asia.* Princeton, New Jersey: Princeton University Press, 1974.

McKhann, Charles F. "The Naxi and the Nationalities Question," in Stevan Harrell, ed. *Cultural Encounters on China's Ethnic Frontiers.* Seattle: University of Washington Press, 1995, 39–62.

Mclean, Fitzroy. *Eastern Approaches.* London: Jonathan Cape, 1949.

McMillen, Donald H. *Chinese Communist Power and Policy in Sinkiang 1949–1977.* Boulder, Colorado: Westview Press, 1979.

————. "Xinjiang and Wang En-mao: New Directions in Power, Policy and Integration," *China Quarterly* 99 (September 1984), 569–593.

Medlin, William K., William M. Cave, and Finley Carpenter. *Education and Development in Central Asia: A Case Study on Social Change in Uzbekistan.* Leiden: E.J. Brill, 1971.

Melby, John F. *The Mandate of Heaven.* London: Chatto and Windus, 1969.

Menges, Karl H. and Johannes Benzing, "Classification of the Turkic Languages," *Philologiae Turcicae Fundamenta.* Wiesbaden: Apud Franciscum Steiner, 1959, I, 1–10.

————. *The Turkic Languages and Peoples: An Introduction to Turkic Studies.* Wiesbaden: Harrassowitz, 1968.

Millward, James. *Beyond the Pass: Commerce, Ethnicity and the Qing Empire in Xinjiang, 1759–1864.* Unpublished Ph. D. dissertation, Stanford University, 1993.

Mitchell, John. *The Russians in Central Asia: Their Occupation of the Kirghiz Steppe and the Line of Syr-Daria.* London: E. Stanford.

Miyawaki, Junko. "Did a Dzungar Khanate Really Exist?" *Journal of the Anglo-Mongolian Society* 10:1 (1987), 1–5.

Mori-Kazak Autonomous County Survey Compilation Committee, *Mulei-Hasake zizhixian gaikuang* [A Survey of the Mori-Kazak Autonomous County]. Urumqi, Xinjiang: Xinjiang People's Press, 1984.

Morrison, Ian. "Some Notes on the Kazakhs of Sinkiang," *Journal of the Royal Central Asian Society* 36 (1948-49): 67-71.

Moseley, George. *A Sino-Soviet Cultural Frontier: The Ili-Kazakh Autonomous Chou.* Cambridge: East Asian Research Center, Harvard University, 1966.

Murdock, George P. *Ethnographic Atlas.* Pittsburgh: University of Pittsburgh Press, 1987.

————. *Atlas of World Culture.* Pittsburgh: University of Pittsburgh Press, 1981.

————. *Our Primitive Contemporaries.* New York: Macmillan, 1936.

Murzaev, E. M.. *Prirodnye usloviia Sin'tsziana.* [Natural conditions in Xinjiang]. Moscow: Izd-vo Akademii nauk SSSR, 1960.

————. *Prirode Sin'czjana: Formirovanie pustyn' Central'noj Azii* (The Nature of Sinkiang and the Formation of the Deserts of Central Asia). Moscow, 1966. Transl. in JPRS 40299 (1967).

Myrdal, Jan. *The Silk Road.* London: Victor Gollancz Ltd., 1980.

Nadzhip, E. N. *Modern Uigur.* Transl. D. M. Segal. Moscow, 1971.

Nichols, James. *Minority Nationality Cadres in Communist China.* Unpublished Ph.D. dissertation, Stanford University, 1969.

Norins, Martin R. *Gateway to Asia: Sinkiang Frontier of the Chinese Far West.* New York: The John Day Company, 1944.

Nyman, Lars-Erik. *Great Britain and Chinese, Russian and Japanese Interests in Sinkiang, 1919-1934.* Stockholm: Esselte Studium, 1977.

Olcott, Martha Brill. *Kazakhs.* Stanford, California: Stanford University Press, 1987; 1995.

————. *Central Asia's New States.* Washington, D.C.: US Institute of Peace Press, 1996.

Oraltay, Hasan, *Kazak Türkleri* [The Kazak Turks]. Istanbul: Türk Kültür Yayini, 1961.

————. *Alas: Turkistan Milli Istiklal Parolasi* [Alash: The Rallying Cry of the Turkestani Turks National Indpendence]. Istanbul: Buyuk Turkeli Yayinlari, 1973.

Peissel, Michel. *Cavaliers of Khan: The Secret War in Tibet.* London: William Heineman Ltd., 1972.

Price, M. Phillip. "The Great Kazakh Epic," *Journal of the Royal Central Asian Society* 41 (1954), 249-52.

Prouty, L. Fletcher. *The Secret Team: The CIA and Its Allies in Control of the United States and the World.* Englewood Cliffs, New Jersey: Prentice Hall Inc., 1973.

Prejevalsky, Nikolai [Przheval'skii, Nikolai N.]. *Mongolia, the Tangut Country, and the Solitudes of Northern Tibet.* 2 vols. London: S. Low, Marston, Searle & Rivington, 1876.

——. *Iz'' Zajsana cherez'' Khami v'' Tibet'' i na verkhov'ia Zheltoi rieki* [From Zaysan through Hami into Tibet and the Head-waters of the Yellow River]. St. Petersburg: V. S. Balasheva, 1883.

Quested, R.K.I. *Sino-Russian Relations: A Short History.* London: George Allen & Unwin, 1984.

Radloff, Wilhelm, "Das Ili-Thal in Hochasien und seine Bewohner," *Petermann's Geographische Mitteilungen,* 1866, 88–97.

——. *Aus Sibirien.* 2 vols. Leipzig: T.O. Weigel, 1893.

Rakowska-Harmstone, Teresa. *Russia and Nationalism in Central Asia: The Case of Tadzhikistan.* Baltimore: Johns Hopkins Press, 1970.

Rea, Kenneth W., and John C. Brewer, eds. *The Forgotten Ambassador: The Reports of John Leighton Stuart, 1946-49.* Boulder, Colorado: Westview Press, 1981.

Riasanovsky, Valentin A. *Customary Law of the Nomadic Tribes of Siberia.* Tianjin: n.p. 1938; reprint, Indiana University Press, Uralic-Altaic Series Number 48 (1965).

Rice, Tamara Talbot. *Ancient Arts of Central Asia.* London: Thames and Hudson, 1965.

Ro'i, Yaacov, ed. *The USSR and the Muslim World.* London: George Allen & Unwin, 1984.

Rossabi, Morris. *China and Inner Asia.* London: Thames and Hudson, 1975.

Rosinger, Lawrence K. *The State of Asia.* New York: Alfred A. Knopf, 1951.

Rudelson, Justin. "Uighur Historiography and Uighur Ethnic Nationalism," in Ingvar Svanberg, ed. *Ethnicity, Minorities and Cultural encounters.* Uppsala, Sweden: Uppsala Multiethnic Papers, 1991.

——. *Bones in the Sand: The Struggle to Create Uighur Nationalist Ideologie in Xinjiang, China.* Unpublished Ph.D. dissertation, Harvard University, 1992.

——. *Oasis Identities: Uyghur Nationalism Along China's Silk Road.* New York: Columbia University Press, 1997.

Rupen, Robert A. "The Absorption of Tuva," in Thomas T. Hammond, ed., *The Anatomy of Communist Takeovers.* London: Yale University Press, 1975.

——. *The Mongolian People's Republic.* Stanford: Stanford University Press, 1966.

——. "Peking and the National Minorities" in Frank Trager, ed. *Communist China 1949-69: A Twenty Year Appraisal.* New York: New York University Press, 1970.

Ryasanovsky, Valentin. *Customary Law of the Nomadic Tribes of Siberia.* Bloomington, Indiana: Uralic and Altaic Series, 1965.

Sadri, Roostram. "The Islamic Republic of Eastern Turkestan: A Commemorative Review," *Journal Institute of Muslim Minority Affairs* 5:2 (1984), 194-320.

Saguchi, Toru. "Kazakh Pastoralists on the Tarbaghatai Frontier under the Ch'ing," *Proceedings of the International Conference on China Border Area Studies* (April 23–30, 1984), National Chengchi University, Taipei, Taiwan, 1985, 953–996.

————. "Kazahu dai oruda no shuzoku shudan" [Ethnic Groups of the Great Horde Kazakhs], *Toyoshi kenkyu* 25:2 (1966) 1–34.

Samolin, William. *East Turkestan to the Twelfth Century*. London: Mouton & Co., 1964.

Saunders, J.J. *The History of the Mongol Conquests*. London: Routledge and Kegan Paul, 1971.

Schomberg, Reginald C. F. *Peaks and Plains of Central Asia*. London: Martin Hopkinson Ltd., 1933.

————. "A Fourth Journey in the Tien Shan," *The Geographical Journal* 79:5 (1932), 368-74.

Schwarz, Henry G. *Chinese Politics towards Minorities: An Essay and Documents*. Bellingham: Western Washington State College, 1971.

Seton-Watson, Hugh. *Nations and States*. London: Methuen and Co. Ltd., 1977.

Sharaf Al-zaman Tahir Marvazi. *On China, The Turks and India*. Translated by V. Minorsky. Original Arabic text dated 1120. London: Royal Asiatic Society, 1942.

Sharipzhan, Merhat. "Kazakhs of Eastern Turkestan in Threshold of 21 Century [sic]," *Bitig: Journal of the Turkish World* (January 1997), 18–21.

She, Lingyun, "Yi jingqi qianshe jiu Xinjiang yongjiu heping" [Economic contruction in Xinjiang as a means to secure peace], *Tianshan yuegan* [Tianshan Monthly] 1 (October 15, 1947), 9–15.

Sheridan, James E. *China in Disintegration: The Republican Era in Chinese History, 1912-1949*. London: The Free Press, Collier Macmillan Publishers, 1975.

Shevel, I. B. "Natsional'noe stroitel'stvo v Sin'czianskom Uigurskom Avtonomnon Raione Kitaiskoi Narodnoi Respubliki," [National Reconstruction in the Xinjiang-Uyghur Autonomnous Region of the People's Republic of China]. *Sovetskaia etnografia* 1956:2,

Shieh, Milton J.T. *The Kuomintang: Selected Historical Documents 1894-1969*. New York: St. John's University Press under the auspices of the Center of Asian Studies, 1970.

Shipton, Diana. *The Antique Land*. London: Hodder and Stoughton, 1950.

Sih, Paul K.T. (Hsueh, Kuang-chien). *Nationalist China During the Sino-Japanese War, 1937-1945*. Hicksville, New York: Exposition Press, 1977.

Sinor, Denis, ed. *The Cambridge History of Early Inner Asia*. Cambridge: Cambridge University Press, 1990.

Skrine, Francis Henry and Edward Denison Ross. *The Heart of Asia: A History of Russian Turkestan and the Central Asian Khanates*. London: Methuen and Co., 1899.

Sladovshkii, M. I. *Istoriia torgovo-ekonomicheskikh otnoshenii SSSR s Kitaem, 1917–1974* [History of Trade and Economic Relations between the USSR and China, 1917–1974]. Moscow: Nauka, Glas. red. vostochnai lit-ry, 1977.

Smith, Anthony, D.S. *Nationalism in the Twentieth Century*. Oxford: Martin Robertson, 1979.

Smith, D. Howard. *Chinese Religions*. London: Weldenfeld & Nicolson, 1968.

Smith, Wilfred Cantwell. *Islam in Modern History*. London: Oxford University Press, 1957.

Smock, David R. *The Politics of Pluralism*. New York: Elsevier Press, 1975.

Song, Xilian. *Yingquan jiangjun* [The Falcon and Hound General]. Taipei: Li Ao Press, 1995.

Stein, Aurel. *Innermost Asia: Detailed Report of Exploration in Central Asia, Kan-su and Eastern Iran*. 2 vols. London: Oxford University Press, 1928.

Stein, M.A. *Archaeological Exploration in Chinese Turkestan*. London: Eyre and Spottiswoode, 1901.

————. *On Ancient Central Asian Tracks*. London: Macmillan & Co. Ltd., 1933.

Su, Beihai. *Hasakezu wenhuashi*. [The cultural history of the Kazak Nationality]. Urumqi, Xinjiang: Xinjiang University Press, 1989.

Sullivan, Walter. "Chiefs Vow Fights on Sinkiang Reds," *New York Times*, April 18, 1949.

Sun, Yatsen. *The Principle of Nationalism*. Translated by Frank W. Price. Taipei: China Cultural Service, n.d.

————. *The Three Principles of the People, with Two Supplementary Chapters by Chiang Kaishek*. Taipei: China Publishing Co., n. d.

Svanberg, Ingvar. "Kazakstan and the Kazakhs," in Graham Smith, ed. *The Nationalities Question in the Post-Soviet States*. London: Longman, Inc. 1996.

————. "Xinjiang Kazak Adoption Practices," *Central Asiatic Journal* 38:2 (1994), 235–243.

————. "In Search of a Kazakhstani Identity," *Journal of Area Studies*, 4 (1994), 113–123.

————. "Qazaqtar Turkijaga Qajdan barghan?" *Egemendi Qazaqstan* 21 (1991), 4.

————. "Contemporary Changes among the Kazaks," in Ingvar Svanberg, editor, *Ethnicity, Minorities and Cultural Encounters*. Uppsala, Sweden: Uppsala Multiethnic Papers, 1991.

————. *Kazak Refugees in Turkey*. Uppsala, Sweden: Studia Multiethnica Upsaliensia, 1989.

————. "The Nomadism of Ora Juz Kazaks in Xinjiang 1911–1949," in I. Svanberg and L. Benson, eds. *The Kazaks of China: Essays on an Ethnic Minority*. Uppsala, Sweden: Stu Multietnica Upsaliensia, 1988.

————. *The Altaic-speakers in China: Numbers and Distribution*. Uppsala, Sweden: Multiethnic Papers, 1988.

————. "The Folklore of Teeth among Turkic and Adjacent People," *Central Asiatic Journal* 31:1–2 (1987) 111–137.

————. "Vilken roll spelar den kazakiska diasporan?," in *Centralasien: gamla folk soker ny vag*, eds. Farid Abbaszadegan and Bo Utas. Uppsala: Sallskapet for Asienstudier, 1995, 15–25.

————. "Vad hander i Xinjiang?," *Internationella Studier* 1997:3, 58–71.

Szporluk, Roman, ed. *National Identity and Ethnicity in Russia and the New States of Eurasia*. Armonk, New York: M.E. Sharpe, Inc., 1994.

Tashjean, John E. *Where China Meets Russia: An Analysis of Dr. Starlinger's Theory*. Washington: Central Asian Collectanea, No.2, 1959.

Teichman, Sir Eric. *Journey to Turkistan*. London: Hodder and Stoughton Ltd., 1936.

————. "Chinese Turkestan," *Journal of the Royal Central Asian Society* 23:4 (1936), 561-78.

Temir, Ahmet. "Die nordwestliche Gruppe der Türksprachen," in *Handbuch der*

Orientalistik, ed. Berthold Spuler, Vol. I:5:1. Leiden and Köln: Brill, 1963, 163–173.

Tong, Hollington K., ed. *China Handbook 1937–45 with 1946 Supplement.*. Compiled by the Chinese Ministry of Information. New York: The Macmillan Co., 1947.

Toops, Stanley W. "Tourism in Xinjiang: Practice and Place," in Alan A. Lew and Lawrence Yu, eds. *Tourism in China*. Boulder, Colorado: Westview Press, 1995.

Tsao, Wen-yen, ed. *The Chinese Yearbook 1944-45*. Compiled by the Council of International Affairs, Chungking. Shanghai: The China Daily Tribune Publishing Co., 1946.

Tsao, W.Y. *The Constitutional Structure of Modern China*. Melbourne: Melbourne University Press, 1947.

Tuzmuhamedov, R. *How the National Question Was Solved in Soviet Central Asia (A Reply to Falsifiers)*. Translated by David Fidlon. Moscow: Progress Publishers, 1973.

U.S. Department of State. *Foreign Relations of the United States Diplomatic Papers*: Vol.7 (1945), vol.10 (1946), vol.7 (1947), vol.9 (1948), vol.9 (1949). Washington: U.S. Government Printing Office, 1969.

U.S. Department of State. Records of the Office of Strategic Services, 1942-48. Reports numbered 26051, 35656, 43256, 45670, 48871, 66568, 69604, 103722, 117975, 137188, XL 32642.

U.S. Department of State. Records of the Office of Strategic Services, Research and Analysis Branch, 1942–1947. Reports numbered 340, 751 1223, 2911S, 1921, 3331, 3248, 3247.

U.S. Department of State, Office of Intelligence Research, 1947. Reports numbered 4451 and 4461.

Valikhanov, Chokan Chingisovich. *Sobranie sochinenii*. [Collected works]. 5 vols. Alma-Ata: Izd-vo Akademii nauk Kazakhskoi SSSR.

Valikhanov, M.V., et al. *The Russians in Central Asia*. Transl. John and Robert Mitchell. London: n.p. 1865.

Vansina, Jan. *Oral Tradition as History*. Madison, Wisconsin: University of Wisconsin Press, 1985.

Vladimirov, P.P. *China's Special Area*. Bombay: Allied Publishers, 1974.

Voll, John Obert. *Islam: Continuity and Change in the Modern World*. Syracuse, New York: Syracuse University Press, 1994.

Waley-Cohen, JoAnna. *Exile in Mid-Qing China: Banishment to Xinjiang 1758–1820*. New Haven, Connecticut: Yale University Press, 1991.

Wang, Xianghong, "Xinjiang shaoshu minzu renkou fasheng wenti de tantao" [A discussion of issues in Xinjiang's national minority population expansion], *Xinjiang shehui kexue yanjiu* [Xinjiang Academy of Social Sciences Research] 30 (1986), 1–5.

Wang, Zengyuan, ed. *Xinjiang China*. [English language edition] Urumqi, Xinjiang: Xinjiang People's Press, 1989.

Wang, Zhilai, "Shilun jiefang qian woguo Hasakezu de shehui xingzhi," [A Discussion of Our Country's Kazak Society Before Liberation], *Minzu tuanjie* [Minority Unity] 1 (1963), 30–33.

Warikoo, K.B. "Chinese Turkestan during the Nineteenth Century: A Socio-economic Study," *Central Asian Survey*, 4:3 (1985),

Watson, Francis. *The Frontiers of China*. London: Chatto and Windus, 1966.
Weggel, Oskar. *Xinjiang/Sinkiang. Das zentralasiatische China. Eine Landeskunde*. Hamburg: Institut für Asienkunde, 1984.
Weigert, Hans W. *Generals and Geographers: The Twilight of Geo Politics*. London: Oxford University Press, 1942.
Weiner, Myron. "Peoples and States in a New Ethnic Order," *Third World Quarterly*, 13:2 (1992), 317–333.
Wiens, Harold J. "The Ili Valley as a Geographic Region of Hsin-chiang," *Current Scene* 7:15 (1969), 1-19.
————. "The Historical and Geographical Role of Urumchi, Capital of Chinese Central Asia," *Annals of the Association of American Geographers* 53:4 (1963), 441-64.
Wheeler, Geoffrey. *Racial Problems in Soviet Muslim Asia*. London: Oxford University Press, 1962.
————. *The Peoples of Soviet Central Asia*. London: The Bodley Head, Ltd., 1966.
————. "Nationalism vs. Communism in Asia," *Asian Affairs* 64 (1977), 38-47.
————. "The Muslims of Central Asia," *Problems of Communism* 16:5 (1967), 72-81.
Whiting, Allen S. *Sinkiang: Pawn or Pivot*. East Lansing Michigan: Michigan State University Press, 1958.
Whitson, William W. *The Chinese High Command*. New York: Praeger Publishers Inc., 1973.
Winner, Thomas G. *The Oral Art and Literature of the Kazakhs of Russian Central Asia*. Durham, North Carolina: Duke University Press, 1958.
Winnington, Alan. *Tibet, Record of a Journey*. New York: International Publishers, Inc., 1957.
Winter, Clyde-Ahmed. "Chinese Langauge Policy and the Muslim Minorities in Xinjiang," *Asian Profile*, 10 (1982), 413–419.
Woodhead, H.G.W. *The China Year Book 1934*. Shanghai: The North-China Daily News and Herald, Ltd., 1934.
Wu, Aitchen K. *Turkistan Tumult*. London: Methuen & Co., 1940. Reprinted, Hong Kong: Oxford University Press, 1984.
————. "The Fourteen Peoples of Chinese Turkestan," *Journal of the West China Border Research Society*, 15, series A (1944), 83–93.
Xinjiang Academy of Social Sciences Research Committee, *Xinjiang jianshi* [A concise history of Xinjiang]. 3 vols. Urumqi, Xinjiang: Xinjiang People's Press, 1980.
Xinjiang-Weiwuer zizhiqu difanzhi bianji weiyuanhui [Xinjiang-Uyghur Autonomous Region Gazetteer Editorial Committee]. *Xinjiang nianjian 1992* [Xinjiang Yearbook 1992]. Urumqi: Xinjiang People's Press, 1992.
Xinjiang-Weiwuer zizhiqu difanzhi bianji weiyuanhui [Xinjiang-Uyghur Autonomous Region Gazetteer Editorial Committee]. *Xinjiang nianjian 1995* [Xinjiang Yearbook 1995]. Urumqi: Xinjiang People's Press, 1995.
Xinjiang Production Contruction Corps Historical Records Publication Committee. *Xinjiang shengchan jianshe bingtuan nianjian* [Xinjiang production construction corps yearbook]. Urumqi, Xinjiang: Xinjiang University Press, 1990.
Xinjiang Production Construction Corps Yearbook Compilation Committee.

Xinjiang shengchan jianshe bingtuan tongji nianjian [Statistical Yearbook of Xinjiang Production and Contruction Corps]. Urumqi, Xinjiang: China Statistical Press, 1993.

Xinjiang-Uyghur Autonomous Region General Survey Compilation Committee. *Xinjiang-Weiwuer zizhiqu gaikuang* [A Survey of the Xinjiang-Uyghur Autonomous Region]. Urumqi, Xinjiang: Xinjiang People's Press, 1985.

Xinjiang-Uyghur Autonomous Regional Publications Committee. *Xinjiang tongzhi* [The Complete Records of Xinjiang]. Vol. 24. Urumqi, Xinjiang: Xinjiang People's Press, 1992.

Xu, Xifa, ed. *Zhongguo shaoshu minzu jihua shengyu gailun* [An introduction to China's minority nationalities family planning]. Urumqi, Xinjiang: Xinjiang People's Press, 1995.

Yakolev, A.G. *The Role of the People's Liberation Army in Economic Construction in the Outlying Districts of the Chinese People's Republic in 1950–1955.* Moscow: Kratkuye Sobshcheniya Instituta Vostokevedeniya 21, 1959. Translation and comment in *Central Asian Review*, 5:2 (1957).

Yang, Richard. "Sinkiang under the Administration of Governor Yang Tseng-hsin, 1911–1928," *Central Asiatic Journal* 11:1 (1961), 270–316.

Yu, Maochun. *OSS in China: Prelude to Cold War.* London: Yale University Press, 1996.

Yuan, Tsing. "Yakub Beg (1820–1977) and the Moslem Rebellion in Chinese Turkestan," *Central Asiatic Journal* 11 (1961), 134–167.

Zayir, Sultanov (Caodanuofu Zhayier). *Wujun de geming licheng* [The revolutionary course of the Fifth Army]. Beijing: People's Liberation Army Press, 1989.

Zenkovsky, Serge A. *Pan-Turkism and Islam in Russia.* Cambridge, Mass: Harvard University Press, 1967.

Zhang, Dajun. *Xinjiang jin sishi nian bianluan jilue* [A Record of Xinjiang's Past Forty Years of Turmoil]. Taipei: Zhongyang wenwu gongyingshe,1954.

Zhang, Dajun. *Xinjiang fengbao qishinian* [Seventy Years of Turmoil in Xinjiang]. 12 vols. Taibei: Lanxi chubanshe you xian gongsi, 1980.

Zhang, Zhizhong. *Zhang Zhizhong huiyi lu* [The Memoirs of Zhang Zhizhong] 2 vols. Beijing: Historical Materials Press, 1985.

Zhou, Qing, and Wong, Yu. "A Few points Concerning the Population Growth of China's Minority Nationalities," *Chinese Sociology and Anthropology* 16:3–4 (1984), 184–198.

Index

About the Authors

Linda Benson is professor of history at Oakland University in Rochester, Michigan. She received an M.Phil. from the University of Hong Kong (1976) and her Ph.D. from the University of Leeds (1986), both for research on the Xinjiang region of China. A former resident of Hong Kong, Taiwan, and Great Britain, she has taught in the United States since 1988. In addition to numerous articles on republican-era Xinjiang, she is also the author of *The Ili Rebellion* (1990) and coeditor with Ingvar Svanberg of *The Kazaks of China* (1988).

Ethnologist and author **Ingvar Svanberg** is a research associate in the Department of East European Studies and the Department of History of Religions at Uppsala University, Sweden. He has conducted fieldwork among the Kazaks in Xinjiang and Turkey, as well as among the Kazak diaspora of Germany and Sweden. He has written some fifty books and numerous articles in English and Swedish on a wide range of topics, and he is author of *Kazak Refugees in Turkey* (1989) and *Gypsies (Roma) in the Post-Totalitarian States* (1995), and is coeditor with Linda Benson of *The Kazaks of China* (1988).